PLUMBING

- and -

RENOVATIONS

by Lauri Romanzi, MD

If you have a uterus or know someone who does,
this book is for you

Beauty Call Books
P.O. Box 3437
Church Street Station
New York, NY 10008-3437
www.beautycallbooks.com

LCCN 2008908547
ISBN-10 0-9801903-0-4
ISBN-13 978-0-9801903-0-4
Copyright information available upon request.

Cover Design: Abigail Hart Gray
Interior Design: J. L. Saloff
Illustrations: Michael J. Maddalena, Madd Graphix, Inc.
Photography: Cheryl Fleming
Typography: New Baskerville BT, Adobe Jenson Pro,
Century 725, Arial Narrow

v. 1.0
First Edition, 2009
Printed on acid free paper.

In loving tribute to Zelda,

who taught me how to sew.

Contents

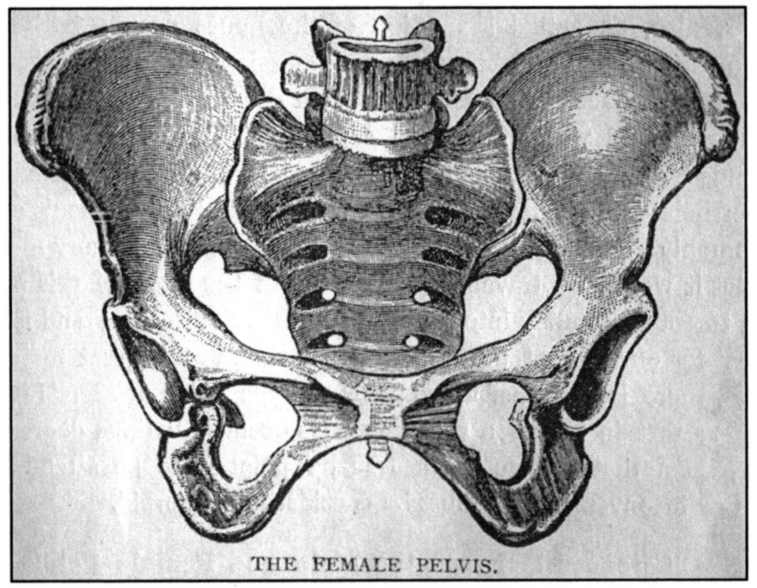

Women's Guide to Health and Happiness, circa 1900

Prologue

I run a clubhouse for big girls, a haven of navel-to-knees magic tricks for women in quest of the ultimate female remedy, vaginal rejuvenation. My specialty, urogynecology, is a hybrid of urology and gynecology that services the "plumbing and renovations" needs of women: plumbing for leaky bladders and bowels, renovations for prolapse, vaginal laxity, fistulas and the like.

Lots of patients think it's something new, this urogynecology specialty, tailor-made for their particular unhappy stew of symptoms. But it's not new at all. Gynecologic remodeling spans the centuries, highlighted by the groundbreaking surgical repair techniques for childbirth-related injuries developed by Dr. J. Marion Sims (1813-1883), the godfather of female pelvic surgery, whose marble bust presides over the New York Academy of Medicine on 103rd Street and Fifth Avenue in the shade of Manhattan's Central Park.

Urogynecology overlaps with its urologic cousin,

the Adam's rib subspecialty dubbed "female urology." Urology, being traditionally concerned with the plumbing of boys, caters to the female half of humanity under this pink ribbon label.

The historical roots vary, with the gynecology more focused on renovations and urology geared toward plumbing. Over the last 20 years special fellowship programs sprouted in both urogynecology and female urology, each churning out doctors skilled in both plumbing and renovations, creating an area of specialty overlap. Similar to rhinoplasty, where patients may avail the services of an ear, nose and throat surgeon or a plastic surgery specialist, or spinal disc procedures, where one chooses between an orthopedic surgeon or a neurosurgeon, urogynecology and female urology intertwine, giving patients a wide selection of pelvic health clinicians. These two new subspecialty labels fit the classic Madison Avenue marketing paradigm of refocusing the eye of the "consumer" on an established but reshuffled, repackaged and relabeled "product", much like the advent of New Coca-Cola in the beverage arena or the relaunching of girdles under the sexy trademark Spanx™. Sexy girdles, who knew?

Call it what you will, the surgical side of vaginal rejuvenation has much in common with fine tailoring. As a girl I spent a lot of time in the company of seamstresses and upholsterers, and I kid you not, as a urogynecologist I use bias tape, the basting stitch, collar facings, upholstery needles, the hem stitch, darning, patches, and the taking in of darts—everything but zippers and buttonholes.

They don't teach vaginal rejuvenation in medical school; it doesn't exist in academic medicine. Not that the medical students aren't curious. They are keenly interested in all things vaginal, as evidenced in my annual anatomy cadaver lab teaching sessions where I am inevitably grilled on the facts and fictions of the anatomically elusive G-spot. Regardless, in three years of medical school, four years of pounding inner-city residency, a reconstructive pelvic surgery fellowship and 20 years of clinical and academic practice, I have yet to come across a lecture, book or course on the topic of "vaginal rejuvenation."

Vaginal rejuvenation, my sisters, is a marketing term, emerging onto the public horizon like a gynecologic freight train, spawning medico-ethical debate among physicians. So great is the angst over this phenomenon that the American College of Obstetrics and Gynecology published a committee opinion in 2007 to clarify its position on the medically undefined procedures of "vaginal rejuvenation," "designer vaginoplasty," "re-virgination" and "G-spot amplification." The directive states that some procedures advertised under these labels may be appropriate for properly selected and counseled patients, but that other procedures, for instance "G-spot amplification," have no historical medical indication and lack data showing that they work and are safe. That's fair. But this understandably vague and limited interpretation of what is and isn't "vaginal rejuvenation" reminds me of the story about blind men defining an elephant, as my colleagues seize upon any one of a number of alleged "rejuvenation" procedures and wail, "Vaginal rejuvenation is a scam foisted upon women in order to promote and profit from genital insecurity," on the one hand to, "Vaginal rejuvenation is the final frontier of post-feminist self-determination," on the other. Completely nutty! From the ridiculous to the sublime, vaginal rejuvenation is a word pair with an impact unlike any other in the recent history of gynecology.

Civilians, blissfully unaware of the ongoing medical food fight over whether or not they are being duped into surgery that they "don't really need," *love* the term vaginal rejuvenation. What a great idea! But what is it? In my experience, each woman brings to the consultation desk her own unique mix of expectations that often extends well beyond the "plastic alteration and sexual enhancement" procedures currently advertised under the "rejuvenation label." Here's what my patients tell me they're looking to make-like-new:

Patient Definitions of Vaginal Rejuvenation

- Vaginal muscle fitness
- Lift a dropped bladder
- Tighten a wide-open vagina
- Restore the hymen
- Fix a bulging rectum
- Repair a leaky bladder
- Recontour uneven or extra long labia
- Restore anal control
- Lift a dropped uterus

None, not a single one, of these procedures is new. Seriously, it's all been available for decades, some of it for hundreds of years, tucked away deep in the gynecologic book of magic, made accessible to only the most injured of women at the sole discretion of the physician. Here is the list with the medical labels:

Vaginal Rejuvenation	Traditional Medical Terminology
Vaginal muscle fitness	Pelvic Floor Rehabilitation
Lift a dropped bladder	Anterior Colporrhaphy
Tighten a wide vagina	Perineoplasty
Restore the hymen	Hymenoplasty
Fix a bulging rectum	Posterior Colporrhaphy
Repair a leaky bladder	Urethral Sling
Recontour labia	Labiaplasty
Restore anal control	Anal Sphincteroplasty
Lift a dropped uterus	Uterine Resuspension, aka. Hysteropexy

So, if none of these procedures are new, why are doctors dickering over the term vaginal rejuvenation? It's the label that's the culprit here, along with a couple of the more controversial procedures. The most debated operations are labiaplasty, G-spot amplification, clitoral unhooding, and hymen restoration, the first being cosmetic and the last typically (but, increasingly, not always) sought by women from cultural backgrounds that mandate virginity on the honeymoon mattress. G-spot amplification (collagen injection into the anterior vaginal wall at the G-spot) and its emerging cousin, subclitoral hyaluronic acid injection, (hyaluronic acid is a facial filler for wrinkles) are both alleged to enhance sexual pleasure, although neither have a smidge of data showing that this is indeed true, nor any evidence that either procedure is safe. These two sexual enhancement procedures are sure to spark continued debate. Neither labiaplasty, hymen restoration or perineoplasty are new, however, and none commanded dueling repartee in the medical journals before the advent of the term vaginal rejuvenation, a patient-oriented phrase held aloft by a growing demand that is foreign to classic gynecologic training.

In the past these therapies were doled out almost as an afterthought, and then only if the patient suffered miserable symptoms. Women crept about in consultation after consultation, looking for someone to help them with "that bulge down there," or explain why they dribble urine on the tennis court, or to figure out why neither they nor their husbands were feeling any contact during sex. The quest for a sympathetic clinician often required Herculean levels of tenacity and resilience.

This white-coat wall of indifference is toppling fast. Women, enlightened by this new vaginal rejuvenation label, now actively seek these procedures much earlier and for less severe symptoms than did past generations. This consumer movement is well-timed, riding the ripple effect from the natural birthing movement of the '70s and '80s that set the stage for women to exert more control over their obstetric and gynecologic fates. Trust me, the blooming interest in vaginal rejuvenation is a most unnerving pink elephant on the coffee table of gynecologic traditionalists, schooled in the art of controlling women's health, and not at all prepared to triage patients walking through the door saying, "fix my parts!"

Our mothers and grandmothers and the generations before them were a stoic bunch: vagina wide open like a mayonnaise jar, bladder bulging out with every lift of a grocery bag, straining red in the face to have a bowel movement, urine squirting with every cough and sneeze—they just dealt with it. And when they did come forward, more than likely the response was not, "So, you're not feeling the penis during sex since you had the baby; how dreadful! Let's get you back to normal with a perineoplasty," or, "You've stopped going to the gym because you're afraid you smell of urine? Well, let's strengthen your vaginal muscles with pelvic floor physical therapy and take a look at your dietary and toileting habits. If that doesn't work, we'll talk about whether a sling operation is a good idea for you," but more likely, "You're normal; there's no problem here," or, "You've had a couple of kids; what can you expect?" or, "Go buy some incontinence pads in the drugstore and do more Kegel exercises. See you next year." No joke, women sit across my desk, regaling me with the frustration of being on the receiving end of such dismissive responses at least once a month, today, in the 21st century, in the U.S. of A.

Now why should it be so hard to get a tune-up if you want one? Why would gynecologists, the specialists sworn to uphold the health and happiness of women, act like a bulging bladder or a wide-open vagina isn't worth fixing? In this girl's opinion, I think it's because gynecologic tradition is all about taking things out: getting the baby out safely, taking the troublesome cyst off the ovary, hysterectomy to remove a problematical uterus, tying the tubes, carving out debilitating endometriosis, snipping out troublesome polyps, turning the pelvis into a hollow canyon to root out cancer, and not really about reconstruction. Other specialties, like orthopedics and plastic surgery, understand the notion of reconstruction; it's what they do every day. But in gynecology, the important work is all about REMOVAL of distressing bits and parts. Demolition, yes, restoration, not so much.

But you can have a tune-up, and you don't have to whack out your organs to do it.

In this volume of *Beauty Call* you'll get the inside

scoop on the central reconstructive pelvic procedures, a gynecologic primer, if you will, for women looking to restore their core to a snug, youthful condition. We begin center stage in the gynecologic universe, the vagina.

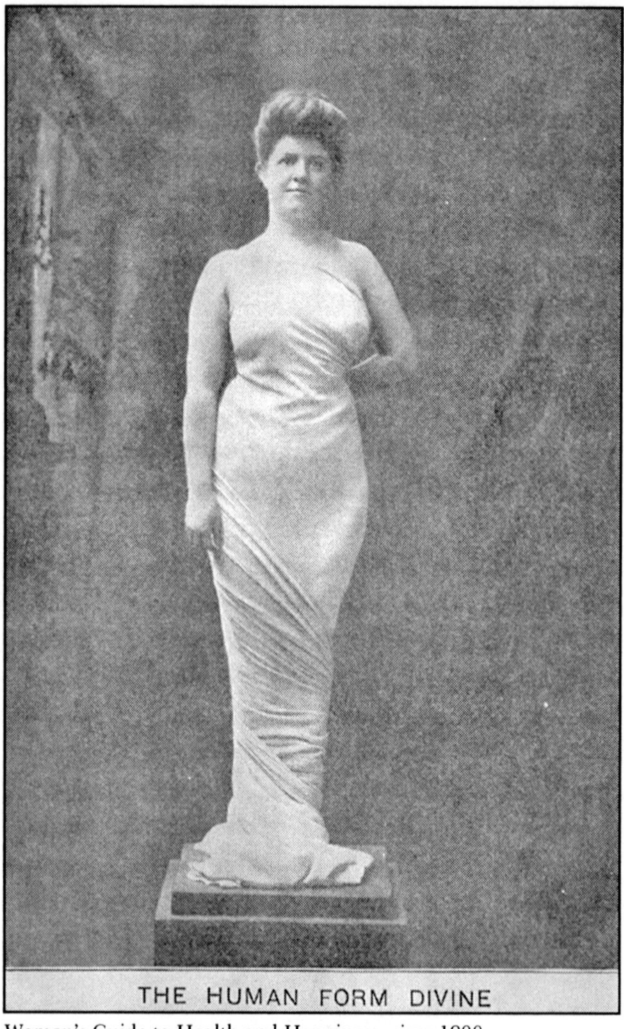
THE HUMAN FORM DIVINE

Women's Guide to Health and Happiness, circa 1900

ONE

Best Room in the House

What's Going on Down There?

A woman's pelvis contains a symphony of body parts surrounded by the Kegel muscles of the Levator Ani (the muscles around the vagina). The uterus drapes gently over the top of the bladder, and the bladder, vagina and rectum are separated from each other by thin elastic walls made of collagen, skin cells and smooth muscle.

The female pelvis houses a three- room cottage, the central room being the vagina, in front of which is the bladder and in back of which is the rectum. The vaginal walls separate each room, the front wall separating the vagina from the bladder and urethra, and the back wall separating vagina from rectum. Above it all, in the central room (the vagina), perches the cervix, the opening to the avocado-shaped uterus, suspended like a chandelier in the ceiling by cables called the uterosacral ligaments.

Below these three rooms sits the perineum, the cornerstone of the basement that separates the vaginal open-

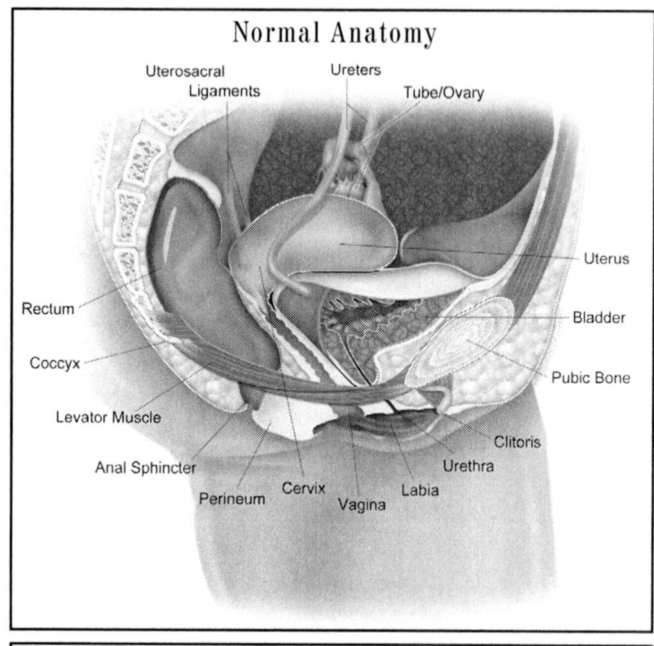

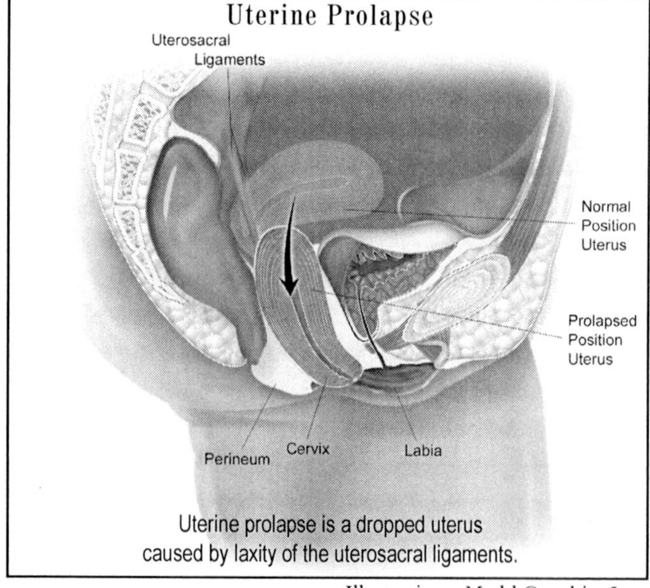

Uterine prolapse is a dropped uterus caused by laxity of the uterosacral ligaments.

Illustrations: Madd Graphix, Inc.

ing from the anus. Around this "house of three rooms" (bladder, vagina, rectum) is a ground-level wraparound terrace of Kegel (levator) muscles.

The walls between the bladder, vagina and rectum sometimes weaken with age and childbirth, causing the bladder to drop, known as a cystocele, or the rectum to bulge, called a rectocele. The connective tissue wedge of the perineum can spread out and thin with childbirth, causing vaginal laxity. And the connective tissue fibers of the uterosacral ligaments can stretch out, letting the uterus prolapse down toward or even out of the vaginal opening.

Chandelier in the Ceiling

When the "cables" (uterosacral ligaments) suspending the "chandelier" (cervix/uterus) in the ceiling of the "center room" (vagina) give way, the chandelier/uterus drops down toward the floor. This condition is called uterine prolapse.

These uterosacral ligaments are to the female pelvis what the ACL (anterior cruciate) ligament is to the knee. They are the main support, and when they go lax instability results in the whole female pelvis. You would think all that ligament stretching is painful, but in most cases there's no pain at all. If your uterus drops, your story might sound like Joan's.

Joan came to me just after the Christmas holidays, worried she may have to forego the planned New Year's family trip to the emerald West Indian island of St. Lucia. Sitting with me one brittle, grey New York City winter's day, her perplexed demeanor reflected her words.

"Something," she told me in urgent tones, "is wrong down there."

With a house full of guests sleeping upstairs on Christmas day, she recounted feeling a pressure deep in her belly that came on suddenly and with little fanfare that morning just as she settled the turkey into the oven. The heaviness lurked the whole day, "Between my tailbone and my groin," nagging her through the hours of basting, baking and tending to guests. Hours later, scurrying to the bathroom just before table seating, her bladder emptied with an unfamiliar, trickling stream. And then she felt it, just above the toilet paper in her hand, a bulge both soft and firm, "Between the lips of my vagina, as if I was giving birth!" She pushed it up painlessly and it came right back down. The first thing that ran through her head was, " Is it cancer?" It wasn't cancer. It was uterine prolapse. Twenty minutes and one pessary later she was back on track with her New Year's family travel plans.

Once the uterus drops down to the level of the vaginal opening you can easily feel your cervix (mouth of the uterus), a firm structure that, should you check yourself with a mirror, looks like a small pink donut in between the labia. It is most often noticeable on the toilet or during strenuous activities like jogging or heavy lifting.

With uterine prolapse you might find that uterine slippage waxes and wanes, not there some days and very obvious, very "out" and bothersome on others. It usually pulls back in when you lie down and is often "in in the morning and out by the evening." It can sometimes cause a low backache in the area of the tailbone.

Front Wall, Back Wall, Wraparound Terrace

Uterine prolapse rarely happens without other pelvic organs dropping down too, its bedfellows being dropped bladder (cystocele), rectal bulge (rectocele), deep pelvic hernia (enterocele) and vaginal laxity (perineal thinning). These different bulges all fall under the umbrella term "Pelvic Organ Prolapse," or POP. Some women have a bit of each, others have only one or two, but whichever and to whatever degree, pelvic organ prolapse is "a woman's hernia."

Cystocele happens when the connective tissue between bladder and vagina wears out or pulls off of the inside of the hip bones, leaving only the vaginal skin to hold up the bladder. The skin of the vagina is too elastic to do the job well and so the bladder bulges down toward the vaginal opening when you stand up, cough, run or lift something.

A similar thinning of connective tissue can occur between rectum and vagina, causing a rectocele. Sometimes there are no symptoms at all, just a bulge. But if it does cause problems, rectocele can make you feel like the vagina is loose during sex, difficulty contracting the vaginal muscles, a bearing-down pressure with strenuous activity, or difficulty passing stool. In fact many women with rectocele will press up on the perineum or backward on the vaginal wall toward the rectum to make bowel movements easier. If you are doing this you may have a rectocele.

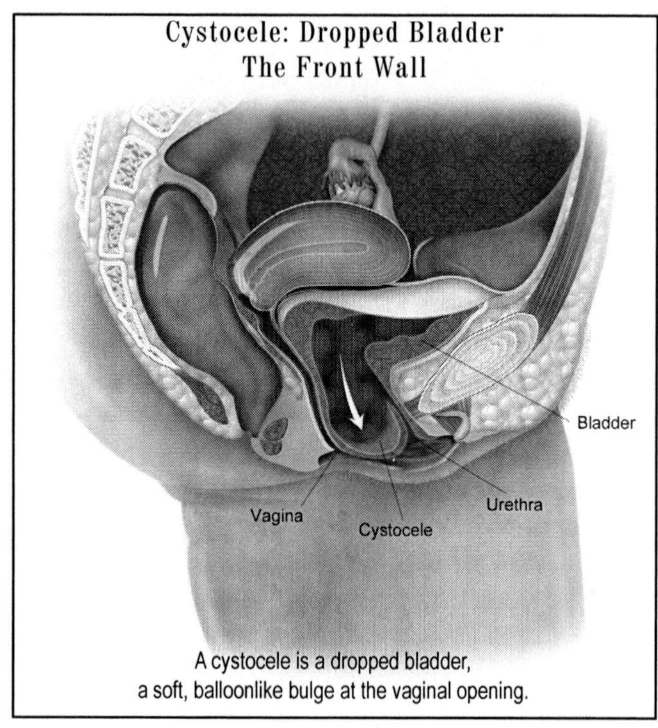

Illustration: Madd Graphix, Inc.

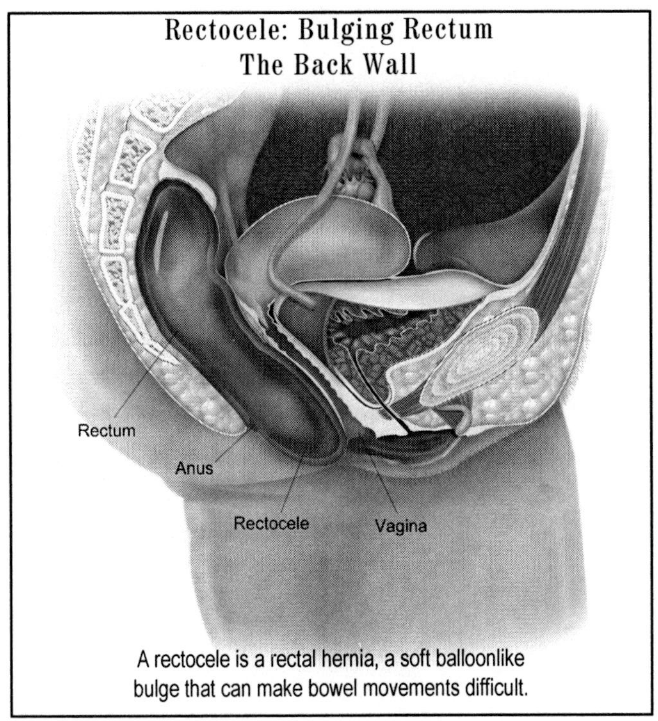

Rectocele: Bulging Rectum
The Back Wall

A rectocele is a rectal hernia, a soft balloonlike bulge that can make bowel movements difficult.

Illustration: Madd Graphix, Inc.

The Cornerstone of the Foundation

The perineum separates the vaginal opening from the anus. The Kegel/levator muscles also connect into the perineum, anchoring it in place. When the connective tissue bundle of the perineum thins out it can make you feel like the vagina is open, or lax, particularly during sex, or during certain exercises like yoga, Pilates™ or jogging. You may do Kegel exercises religiously and still feel the same laxity. You may trap and then pass (very embarrassingly) air from the vagina with certain postures or exercises. This is perineal thinning/vaginal laxity.

The levator (Kegel) muscles surround all of these parts, scaffolding the three rooms (bladder, vagina, rectum) of the pelvis just like a wraparound terrace. Except

Vaginal Laxity: Thin Perineum
The Cornerstone

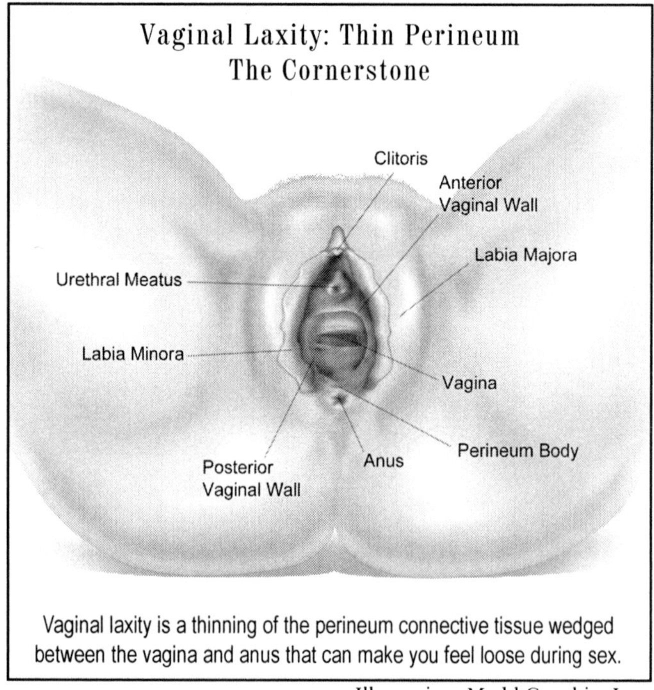

Vaginal laxity is a thinning of the perineum connective tissue wedged between the vagina and anus that can make you feel loose during sex.

Illustration: Madd Graphix, Inc.

this terrace helps hold up the house. In fact, all mammals have this muscle lining the pelvis, men included. In boys the urethra and rectum pass through this muscle complex just like in girls, but of course men have no vagina in the middle of their levator muscles. When men do their Kegel exercises all sorts of things dance about. Next chance you get ask for a demonstration...

Why Me?

Last year I got a call from a graduate student at a nearby Ivy League university looking for help on her thesis paper, the topic of which she kept referring to as "vaginal collapse."

Vaginal collapse was her personal interpretation of pelvic organ prolapse and a reasonable one at that. So we had several long phone chats about the nuts and bolts of pelvic anatomy and the things that can happen to it between being born and passing on. With each call the common thread of her questions made clear that she fully intended to expose the medical misogyny aiding and abetting the collapse of all these vaginas.

I tried to help her, really I did. I gave her statistics, introduced her to research of medical anthropology showing that the same elasticity that allows us to birth children without dying is good for perpetuating the species but not so great for some individuals whose elasticity may lead to prolapse right after or even decades after the baby is born. The graduate student remained steadfast in her conspiracy conviction, insisting I tell her what a woman can do to make sure she never suffers vaginal collapse. Reluctantly I unveiled the honest truth: pelvic organ prolapse is no one's fault, not the women it affects, not the doctors who care for them, not the society we live in, not the toxins in the air. Prolapse started when we first stood up on the African savannah to get a better look at the world. If a woman wants to avoid vaginal collapse the formula is both simple and unfair: never birth babies and die by age 50.

So, if it's no one's fault, why *does* prolapse happen? Pelvic organ prolapse occurs when the collagen fibers in the connective tissues holding up the uterus, bladder, rectum and perineum thin out or stretch. While prolapse is most common in women who have given birth vaginally, it can also happen to women who have never been pregnant or only given birth by Cesarean section.

Connective tissue weakness happens in other areas of the body as well. We all know someone, possibly yourself, who has had physical therapy or surgery for knee or shoulder ligament problems, or an inguinal or belly-button hernia, or a face-lift. All of these reconstructive procedures are done to correct the exact same type of wear and tear connective tissue defects that occur in the female pelvis.

In these other areas of the body connective tissue defects seem less sinister, and if it happens to you chances are you'll roll up your sleeves and do what you have to do to get that body part back into working order. Torn knee ligaments, inguinal hernia, damaged rotator cuff, it's either physical therapy or reconstructive surgery, or both. But, for some reason, when it comes to connective tissue damage in the female pelvis the common response is ... to do nothing. And to blame something. Women often live with severe prolapse for years, believing nothing can be done. They blame themselves, "I never did those Kegel exercises." Or someone else, "My last baby came out so fast right in the bed. That's why my uterus dropped," or, "I had an episiotomy," or, "I didn't have an episiotomy." Many are convinced that the prolapse "Should not be happening to me; I eat right and exercise all the time with my personal trainer; I'm in great shape!"

It is none of those things so don't waste energy on the blame game. Pelvic organ prolapse is just the same as all other wear-and-tear conditions; a little bit of nature and a little bit of nurture. If your connective tissue is extra-elastic (Are you double-jointed or can you do splits with no problem?), if you birth children, if you work hard, play harder and live long enough, you might develop prolapse.

Pelvic organ prolapse affects 30% of all women and half of women who have borne children. One in nine women will have prolapse severe enough to warrant reconstructive surgery in the course of her lifetime. Women over age 80 are the fastest growing segment of North American populations, living far more active lives than preceding generations. This population bubble with its high energy lifestyle is expected to drive a growth in demand for prolapse healthcare services that will be double the rate of population growth over the next three decades. Our great-grandmothers bore this condition with stoicism and modesty; our mothers and sisters are far more likely to seek help.

As with most hernias and ligament tears, prolapse is more likely to happen to you as you get older, whether you stay in shape or never exercise at all, because all connective tissue regenerates more slowly and with less strength in older people than in younger people. But when it comes to women and vaginal prolapse, a growing body of research yields some fascinating explanations as to why some women can birth many children with no prolapse whatsoever while other womens bladders drop after the very first baby is born. Medical data show that women with prolapse may be genetically predisposed, resulting in prolapse clusters among families. Prolapse is associated with altered proportions of collagen (connective tissue), Type I vs. Type III, and biochemical differences in the enzymes that control collagen regeneration and the receptors that regulate hormone activity compared to women without prolapse. The childless sisters of mothers with prolapse are more prone to symptom-free minimal prolapse compared to women whose sisters don't have prolapse. And the second factor in this nature vs. nurture paradigm is childbirth. Big babies and long labors make a woman more prone to pelvic floor disorders. In other words, women who are superelastic are prone to prolapse,

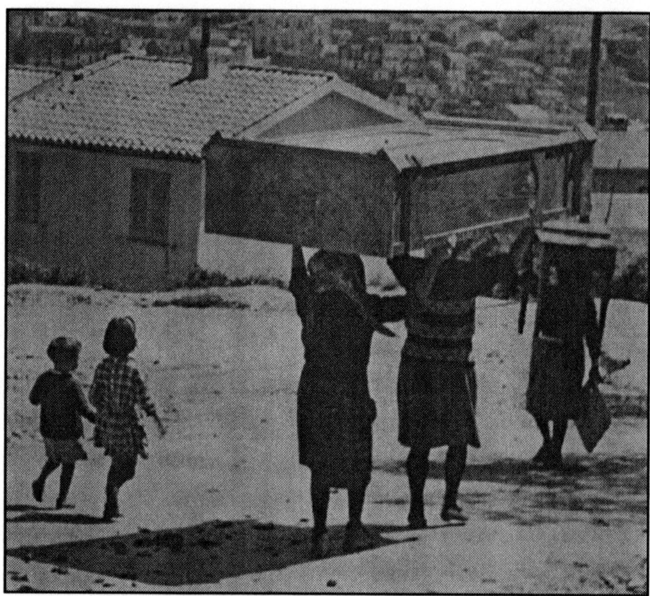

Women of the Shadows by Ann Cornelison, used with permission.

particularly if they give birth to large babies with long labors.

Seat of the Soul

Ask any 10 doctors what to do if the uterus prolapses and 9.7 of them will tell you "Hysterectomy!" This is wrong. If you have uterine prolapse you need the prolapse fixed, not the uterus cut out.

I am a longtime fan of the uterus. I like mine just fine and hope to exit this life with my uterus in tow, not left behind on some pathology department shelf lined with pickled body parts. My guardianship of the uterus materialized during a medical school lecture one day when, mesmerized by the urgent, clipped expectorations of a visiting British nephrologist (kidney specialist), I, circumspect student, sat with note-taking fingers frozen in disbelief, unwilling, yes unable even, to transcribe the proclamation, "The kidney, my dear fledglings, is the seat of the soul!" Since I knew in that instant, as has been my rare privilege to know anything with such certitude, that this poor professor of grand conviction was oh so wrong.

The seat of the soul is not the bladder's filtering cousin, but the uterus, the womb, where one's refuge is always at the ready in recitation of the Hail Mary, "And blessed is the fruit of thy womb, Jesus...," the seat of Adam's soul upholstered in the haven of Eve's skeletal pelvis, revealed in the ruminations of our beloved Shakespeare in *Loves Labours Lost.*

"From women's eyes this doctrine I derive.
They sparkle still the right Promethean fire;
They are the books, the arts, the academes,
That show, contain, and nourish all the world..."

"They sparkle still the right Promethean fire..."

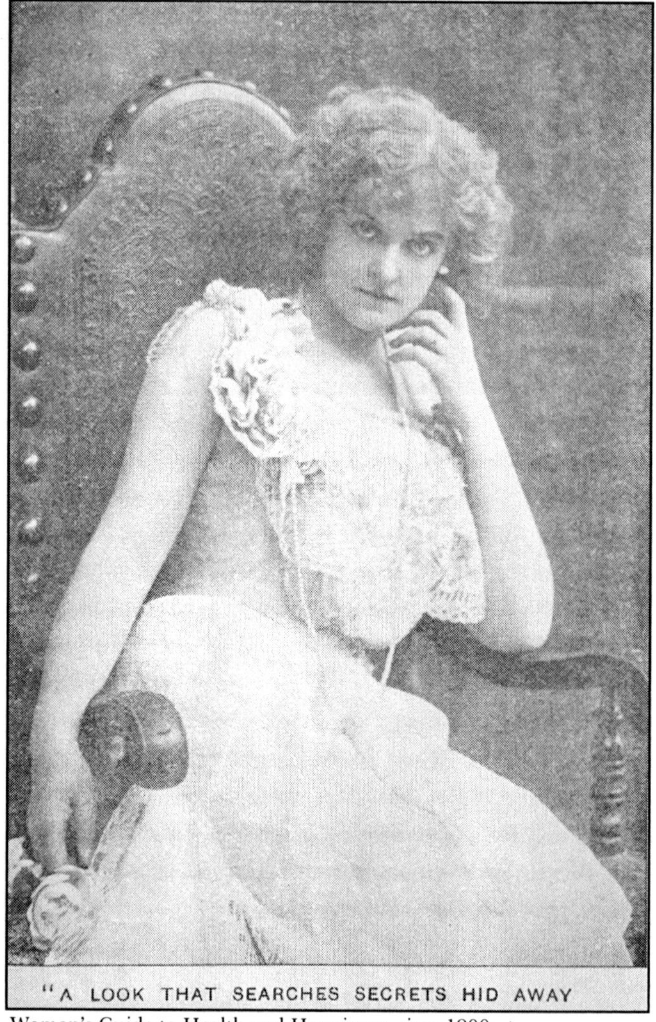
"A LOOK THAT SEARCHES SECRETS HID AWAY

Women's Guide to Health and Happiness, circa 1900

The soul's sparkling Promethean fire may be reflected in the eyes of the gentler sex, but it resides, my friends, in the uterus. Make no mistake.

In flagrant perpetuation of man's inhumanity to man[1] this homeland of the human soul is the most frequently excised organ in the female body. Every year in America, "over 600,000 (hysterectomies) are done. One in three women in the United States has had hysterectomy by age 60."[2]

We see it all the time in the anatomy lab at the medical school where the students learn about human body structure from head to toe on cadavers (preserved dead bodies). When it comes time to learn female pelvic anatomy, the students scramble from table to table looking for the few female cadavers that still have a uterus and ovaries. Most female cadavers are missing there internal organs of procreation and so the students turn to pictures, videos and plastic models. The male cadavers, with rare exception, suffer no such fate, typically exiting this life with penis and testicles intact, in stark contrast to their female counterparts who most often land on the metal dissecting tables fully castrated, vagina ending in a blind pouch, crowned by nothing more than a few loops of bowel.

In the name of health we give every impression of waging war on the uterus, lopping it out as some unnecessary and troublemaking appendage. Before I rouse your radical reflexes to a furious lather however, let's be clear—hysterectomy is not all bad. In cases of life-threatening or recalcitrant uterine conditions, hysterectomy is essential.

1 Robert Burns, Poet Laureate of Scotland, said, "'Mans inhumanity to man makes countless thousands mourn..." (Man Was Made to Mourn)

2 www.4woman.gov/faq/hysterectomy

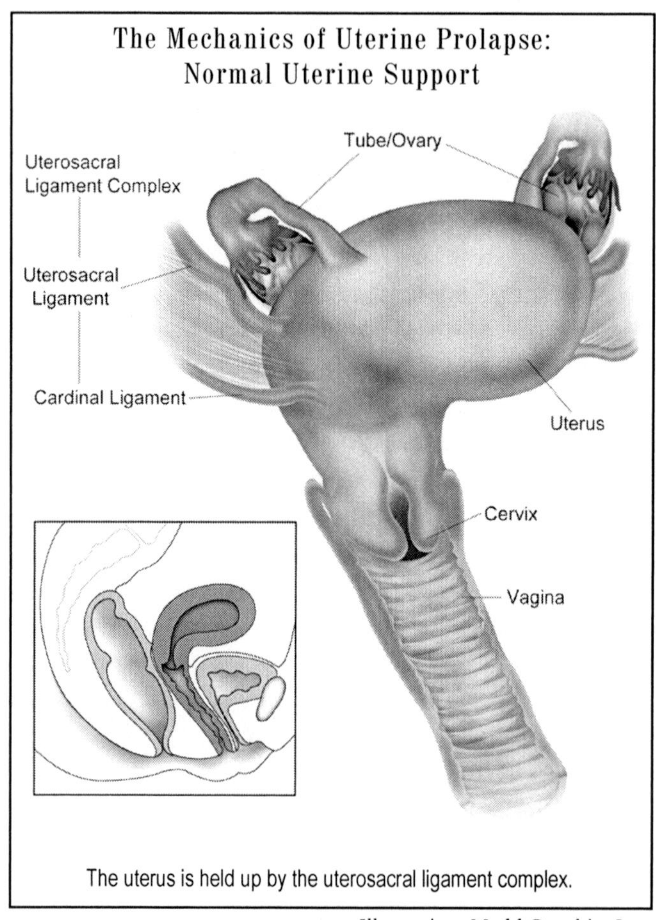

The uterus is held up by the uterosacral ligament complex.

Illustration: Madd Graphix, Inc.

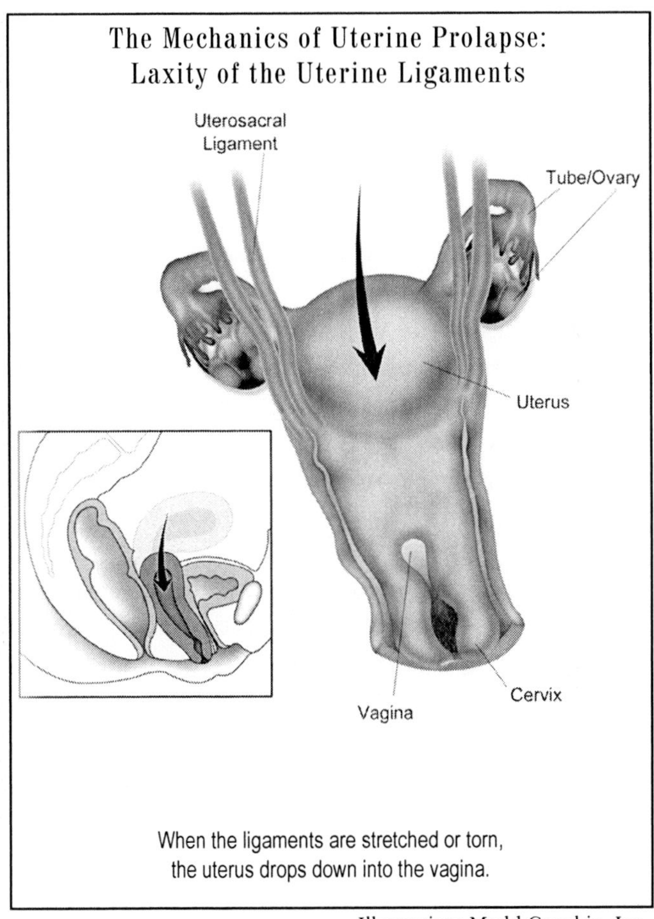

Illustration: Madd Graphix, Inc.

Unfortunately, in many cases the uterus is removed before alternatives are tried, or worse, even considered.

Hysterectomy is a good and wise therapy for women with overwhelming conditions, such as fibroids that refuse to behave despite trying every nonsurgical alternative or hemorrhagic, constant vaginal bleeding from adenomyosis, or the only option in cases of cervical, uterine, or ovarian cancer. These are among the most common and bona fide reasons to remove a uterus. In such instances the hysterectomy is a necessity that will greatly improve, or literally save, the woman's life.

For some bizarre reason, uterine prolapse remains engraved on this list of must-do-hysterectomy rules. This is ridiculous and wrong. You don't have to take out the uterus when it falls. You can lift it up, or "resuspend" it. I repeat: When the uterus drops you can pick it back up. The surgery holds up just as well. You don't have to lose your womb.

Taking out the uterus to fix a prolapse is like taking off the knee cap to fix a torn ligament. Imagine all those knees without knee caps, removed because the knee cap was in the way of the ligament that needed fixing. That is how much sense it makes to lop off a prolapsed uterus just because the ligaments that hold it in place gave way. Either way, uterus in or out, your surgeon must fix those ligaments. If your surgeon tells you there is no way to fix your prolapse without taking the uterus out, or doesn't seem to understand that "IT'S THE LIGAMENTS, STUPID," I advise you to RUN, do not walk, to a second opinion.

Other organs can prolapse too, you know. Like the bladder. It's not at all uncommon for the bladder to drop. You probably know someone whose bladder has dropped.

Chances are she'll never tell you, but she's there, happens all the time. So what do we, the surgeons, do when the bladder drops? Do we say, "Oh my, if the bladder fell once, it could fall again! I know, let's take it out!" No, we do not. We fix the connective tissue and ligament laxities that let that poor bladder hang low and lift it back up.

And the rectum. The rectum can herniate too, bulging into the vagina and making it damned difficult to defecate. Sometimes so difficult that the woman will literally put her thumb into the vagina and push backwards on the bulge in order to poop, a handy maneuver we in medicine call "splinting." And when a despairing, splinting woman shows up with a bulging rectum do we take the rectum out and give her a colostomy? No, we do not. We fix the connective tissue and ligament laxities and restore the position of the poor rectum back to normal, sending the happy patient on her way to a future without her thumb in her vagina.

But when the uterus drops, ah yes, when the uterus drops my friends, the mad irony of a typical dialogue befits a Marx Brothers skit.

> *"Doctor, oh, Doctor, my uterus has dropped!"*
>
> *"Indeed, it has. Let's take it out!"*
>
> *"Oh Doctor, must we?"*
>
> *"But of course, Duchess, why can't you see? If we don't take it out when we operate, it will fall right back down again. Besides, you're not going to have any more children. What do you need it for? It might give you cancer some day you know..."*

"Oh, no! Doctor, I don't want to get cancer! But wait; what about sex? I've heard rumors. My neighbor had a hysterectomy and her sex life was never the same."

"Ah, my dear, the miracles of modern medical research reassure me that all is well here. Your sex life will be just the same or even better without that pesky prolapsed part in the way. Trust me, I have data!"

These common threads of doctor-patient discourse on the topic of uterine prolapse leave many a woman perplexed by this focus on removing the uterus and doubtful of the presumed benefits. With increasing frequency they are leaving their doctor's office with uterus intact, wondering what else can be done to fix the prolapse. What else can be done is PLENTY. What else can be done is on these pages. The fallen uterus is a victim, not a perpetrator, and deserves to be rescued, not stricken from the body to which it belongs. Like good Girl Scouts you must be prepared. The uterus you save may be your own.

There are only two options for treating severe prolapse: surgery or pessary. Pessaries are nifty vaginal widgets that hold prolapse in place. It's sort of like wearing a brace or wrap when your knee ligaments are wobbly, or a truss for inguinal, scrotal or abdominal hernias. Pessaries don't repair the prolapse, but they are easy to use and make you feel and function like normal when they fit well.

Surgery, on the other hand, actually repairs the prolapse; after reconstruction you won't need a pessary ,and you will function and feel much as you did before your first pregnancy. Just like all other reconstructive operations (knee ligaments, hernia repairs, shoulder surgery, face-lifts), there may be complications or less-than-perfect results. In medicine, complications and less-than-perfect results are called risks. All operations, big and small, have risks. Deciding which option (pessary or surgery) fits you best is a lot easier when you have a clear vision of the choices, benefits and risks at hand.

Every year in the United States 200,000 women undergo surgery for prolapse. In most instances hysterectomy is recommended, especially when uterine prolapse is part of the problem. This hysterectomy requirement comes as a shock to many women with prolapse. I hear this in my office all the time. "My bladder dropped and I've been living with this bulge for 5 years. I've been to 7 different doctors and they all insisted that I must have a hysterectomy and I just don't want one." Or, "I just want to get rid of the bulge and not wet my pants at the gym. Why do I have to take the uterus out? There's nothing wrong with it!" These stories of reluctance represent a new and justified trend in gynecologic America.

In fact, there is no scientific data at all that proves that hysterectomy is the best way to fix prolapse.Yet in this country and much of the world at large, hysterectomy continues to serve as the standard surgical technique for this condition. This hysterectomy tradition is increasingly scrutinized by the women it serves, as well it should be, because it is possible to avoid hysterectomy by resuspending a prolapsed uterus with the same if not better results than when the uterus is removed. If you are one of these women, the operation you are looking for is called uterine resuspension or its synonym, hysteropexy. It is safe, effective and minimally invasive.

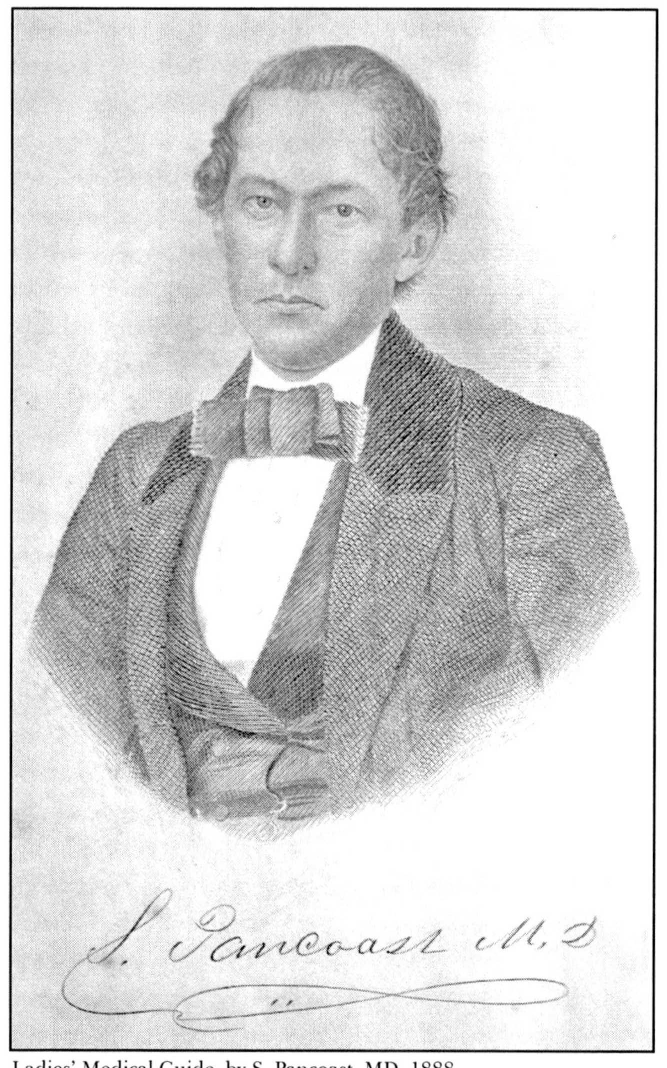

Ladies' Medical Guide, by S. Pancoast, MD, 1888

TWO

Remedies

The Pancoast Perspective

Prolapse has been a part of the human experience for all recorded history, with references found in writings of all eras. From biblical times through the first half of the 20th century remedies and cures remained largely unchanged, reflected in the "Prolapsus" section of Dr. Pancoast's *Ladies' Medical Guide* (1888).

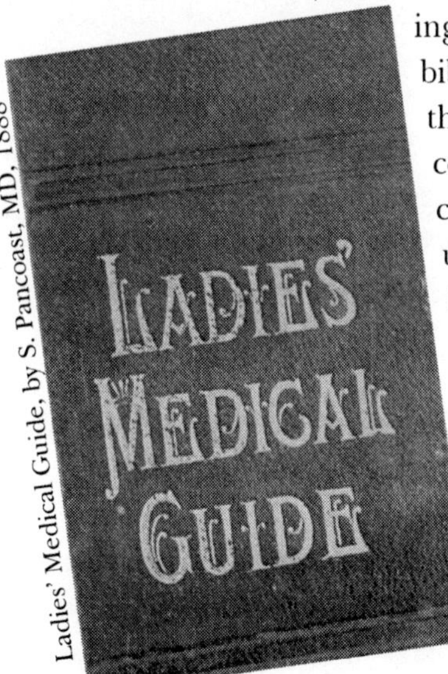

Ladies' Medical Guide, by S. Pancoast, MD, 1888

Such guides to feminine (and masculine) health abounded in the 1800s and early 1900s in prescient tribute to the then-current focus on preventive health and gender-specific medicine.

Our dear Dr. Pancoast laboriously details the symptoms of prolapse from headaches and "a distressed countenance" to palpitations, dyspepsia and a "sensation of weight in the pelvis and groin, at times ... so great that the patient imagines 'everything is dropping through.'"

Dr. Pancoast reveals the working theories of prolapse of that time, some not far flung from our own, including exercising too early after childbearing, dancing, leaping and jumping during menstruation, and abdominal muscle laxity causing the intestines to press down on the womb. His favorite treatment is a properly fitted abdominal binder, followed by admonishments advocating the strict avoidance of corsets, a Victorian-era Catch-22. Cold baths followed by cold water injections into the vagina "must not be omitted", along with "observing the recumbent position as much as possible," and avoiding fatigue. The pessary, made of "silver, gold, wood, cork, sponge and glass," is considered, the use of which he "utterly reprobates" as being "merely palliative at best, while they often produce irritation and inflammation of the os-uteri and vagina, and, by consequence, lay the foundation of more formidable diseases, such as ulceration and cancer of the womb," whereby he proceeds with a hearty endorsement of the use of the "galvanic battery" for prolapse treatment.

Pessaries out, avoiding upright postures, cold water douching and the galvanic battery in. Hmmmm.

In this pre-anesthetic era of the late 1800's, where surgery was reserved for dire emergencies such as a gangrenous leg, rotting tumor or ruptured appendix, we witness in this and similar texts the absence of surgical repair in the treatment options for prolapse. Across the Atlantic in Manchester England the first standardized procedure for prolapse was just being introduced in 1888, the same year Dr. Pancoast published his *Ladies' Medical Guide*. This uterine resuspension technique, called the Manchester-Fothergill operation, is in use even today. Dr. Pancoast and his American colleagues were not aware of, or were aware but not inclined to endorse, the groundbreaking techniques of their British colleagues. To prepare for the future, look to the past.

New, Revised, and Enlarged Subscription Edition.

THE

Ladies' Medical Guide:

An Instructor, Counsellor, and Friend,

Indispensable to Mothers and Daughters.

EMBRACING

A Full and Exhaustive Description of the Structure and Functions of the Reproductive Organs; Anatomy and Physical Perfection of Females, with Diseases of Women and Children, their Causes, Symptoms, and Treatment; the Toilet, Beauty, and Longevity of Females; Startling Facts in Plain Words, etc., etc.

Illustrated by Over One Hundred Accurate Engravings.

BY S. PANCOAST, M.D.,

Professor of Microscopic Anatomy, Physiology, and the Institute of Medicine in Penn Medica University, Philadelphia. Author of "Curability of Consumption," "The Kabbala" "Bright's Disease and its Treatment," etc., etc.

TO WHICH IS ADDED

The Hygiene and Care of Children and the Aged; Care of the Teeth, Eyes, Ears, Skin, Hands, and Feet Early Rising, Exercise, Tabulated Matter, Etc., Etc.

BY C. C. VANDERBECK, M.D., PH.D.,

Lecturer on Hygiene in the Wagner Institute of Science. Member of Victoria Institute, England. Contributor to "The Modern Family Physician," etc., etc.

PHILADELPHIA:

S. I. BELL & COMPANY.

1888.

Ladies' Medical Guide, by S. Pancoast, MD, 1888

TO

THE MOTHERS AND DAUGHTERS

OF THE

UNITED STATES OF AMERICA,

THIS

INSTRUCTIVE TREATISE

ON THE

STRUCTURE AND FUNCTIONS OF THE REPRODUCTIVE ORGANS, DISEASES OF FEMALES AND CHILDREN,

THE TOILET, ETC.,

SCIENTIFICALLY CONSIDERED IN REFERENCE TO

HEALTH BEAUTY AND LONGEVITY:

UNDERTAKEN AT THE SUGGESTION OF MANY LADIES

AND

PROMOTED BY THEIR ENCOURAGEMENT:

IS MOST

RESPECTFULLY INSCRIBED,

BY THEIR SINCERE FRIENDS AND WELL WISHERS.

THE AUTHORS.

(iii)

Ladies' Medical Guide, by S. Pancoast, MD, 1888

Fig. 69.
THE WELL-DEVELOPED, SYMMETRICAL, AND HEALTHY FORM. (From Banning.)

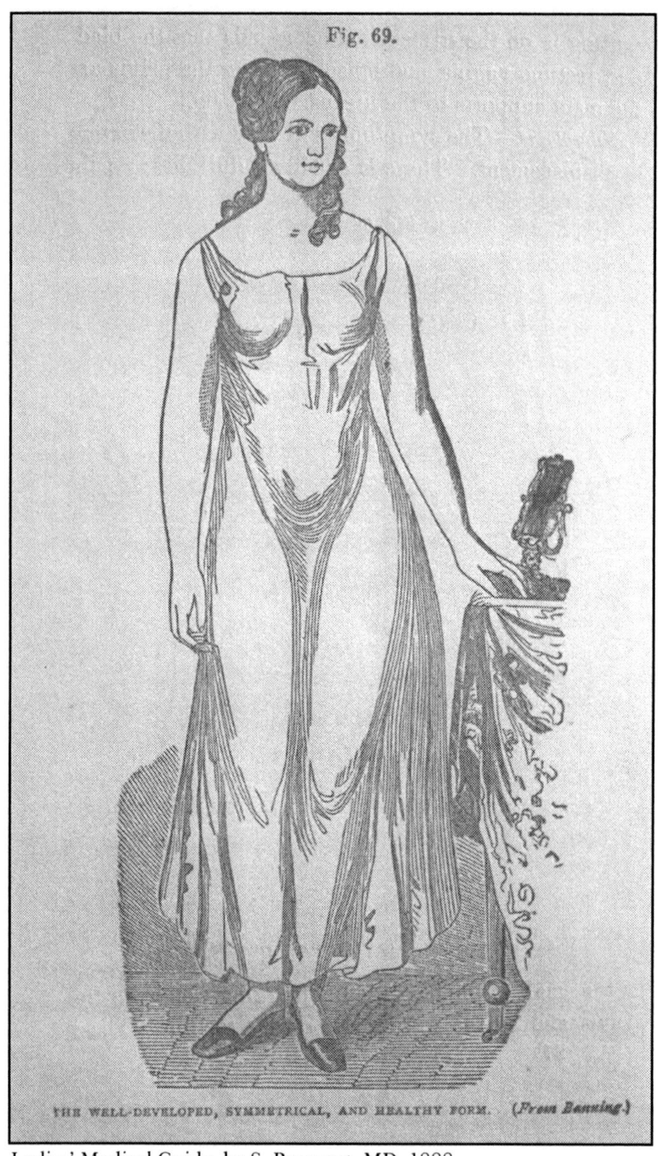

Ladies' Medical Guide, by S. Pancoast, MD, 1888

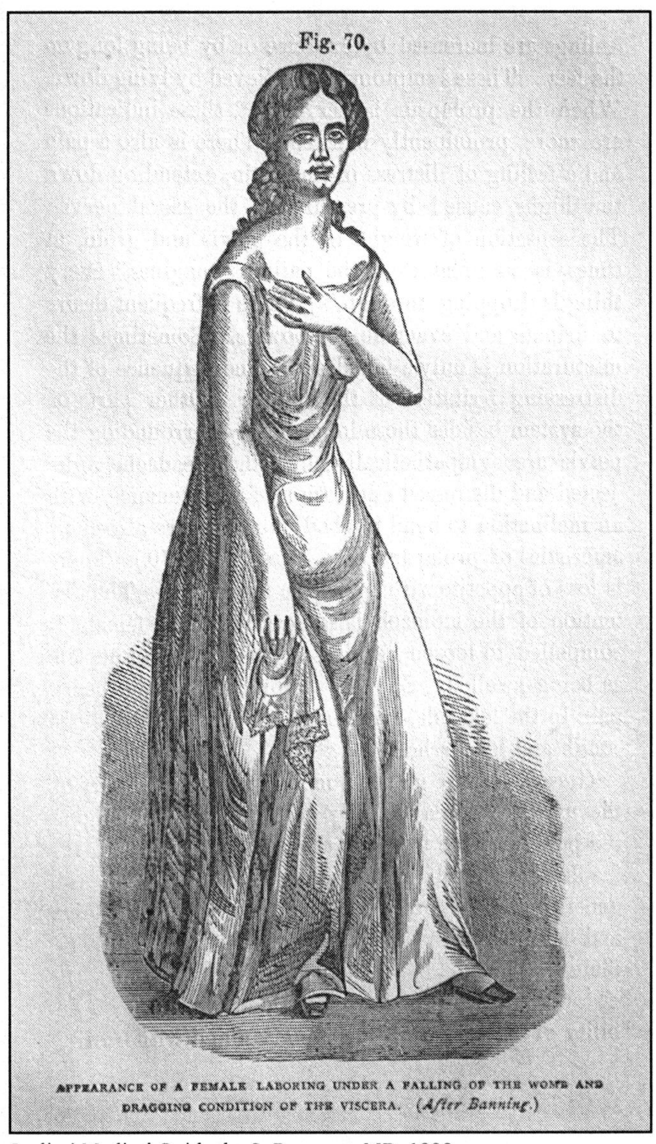

Appearance of a female laboring under a falling of the womb and dragging condition of the viscera. (*After Banning.*)

Ladies' Medical Guide, by S. Pancoast, MD, 1888

℞ Bin. Iodide mercury, ...gr. .
Iodide potash, ...ʒ iij.
Simple syrup, ...℥ iv.
Dose—One teaspoonful three times a day, in water.

In connection with this treatment the patient will require a moderate amount of exercise in the open air, with a rich stimulating diet, while the cold and tepid hip-baths should not be neglected. Sexual intercourse must be strictly avoided, and only moderately indulged after the subsidence of the disease, or the same condition may be induced.

As leucorrhœa is a disorder that requires a nice discrimination in adopting a proper treatment, it might be well in all cases to apply to some skillful physician for preliminary advice, before undertaking its management.

DIVISION III.

DISEASES OF UTERUS AND FALLOPIAN TUBES.

a. PROLAPSUS, OR FALLING OF THE WOMB.—This is the most common form of displacement. By reference to the second Chapter of this work, the reader will find a succinct description of the four ligaments which are intended as partial support to the uterus in the pelvis. These are called round, broad, utero-sacral and utero-cervical ligaments. The uterus is also partially supported by the vagina, and the relaxation of its walls is always sufficient of itself to cause more or less prolapsus. Dr. *Ashwell* maintains that the ligaments afford but very little protection and support to the womb for this organ may be drawn down without

Ladies' Medical Guide, by S. Pancoast, MD, 1888

PROLAPSUS. 413

putting it on the stretch. He contends that the bladder, rectum vagina and muscles lining the pelvis are the main supports to the uterus. (*Fig.* 68.)

Symptoms.—The symptoms will vary with the extent of displacement. There is usually a dull heavy pain

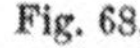

Fig. 68.

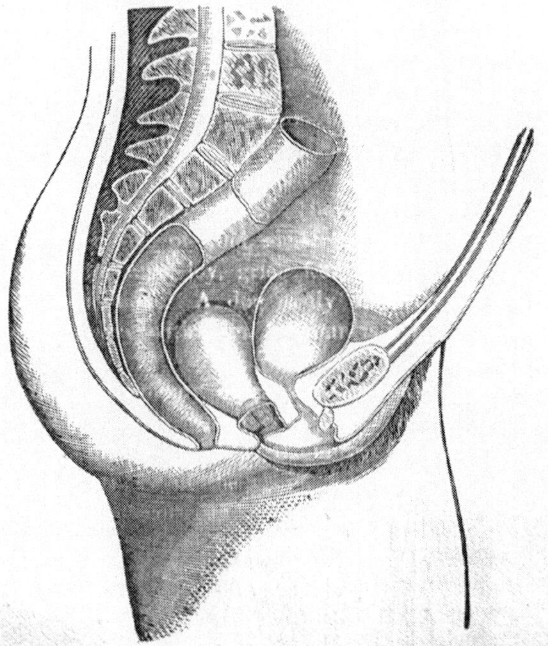

PROLAPSUS OR FALLING OF THE WOMB. (*From Scudder.*)

in the small of the back, and a dragging weight in the pelvis and at the lower part of the rectum. These

27

Ladies' Medical Guide, by S. Pancoast, MD, 1888

416 DISEASES OF FEMALES.

feelings are increased by exercise or by being long on the feet. These symptoms are relieved by lying down. When the prolapsus is very great, these indications are more prominently marked. There is also a pain and a feeling of distress in the groin, extending down the thighs, caused by pressure on the sacral nerves. The sensation of weight in the pelvis and groin, at times, is so great that the patient imagines "every thing is dropping through." There is frequent desire to urinate and evacuate the bowels. Sometimes the micturation is only a few drops, in consequence of the distressing irritation of the bladder. Other parts of the system besides those immediately surrounding the pelvis are sympathetically affected. Headache, a dejected and distressed expression of countenance, with an inclination to bend the body forward, are also characteristics of prolapsus. (See *Figs.* 68 and 70.) There is loss of appetite with dyspeptic symptoms. The distention of the stomach is so great that the female is compelled to loosen her dress. She expresses herself as being swelled. She has palpitation of the heart, pain in the left side, sometimes attended with a slight cough and leucorrhœa.

Causes.—If we glance a moment at the support of the uterus, we may readily perceive that so long as the parts are able to resist the constant action of the diaphragm and abdominal muscles, there cannot, as a general rule, be prolapsus. Whatever tends to relax and debilitate the general system may cause the complaint. The abdominal muscles which support the abdominal viscera are more or less relaxed by a debility of the system. By relaxation and withdrawing

Ladies' Medical Guide, by S. Pancoast, MD, 1888

of support from the abdominal viscera, the bowels are allowed to press upon the pelvic viscera and tissue which support the uterus, and in consequence of this constant pressure it gives way. *Fig.* 71 shows the natural position of the viscera when there is no relaxation of the abdominal muscles, and *Fig.* 72 when there is relaxation and displacement of the womb. Another frequent cause is too early exercise after child bearing. Inflammation of womb, particularly of the cervix, increasing the bulk and weight of the organ, is also a common cause. It is likewise produced by dancing, leaping and jumping, particularly during the period of menstruation, when the organ is naturally increased in weight from the congestion concomitant of the catamenial flow.

Treatment.—First remove the cause. If the abdominal muscles are relaxed, an abdominal supporter is indispensable, in order to support the viscera and take the pressure from the pelvis. Supporters are strongly condemned by some practitioners. Unless they fit properly, they are worse than useless. If properly made, however, they afford great relief, and those accustomed to them cannot be induced to forego their employment.

Supporters have been recommended by manufacturers as applicable to all uterine diseases. Hence the abuse of them has led to their condemnation in toto. If we condemn all good and useful articles because they are liable to be abused, we would soon discover our error. I recommend the supporter in all cases of relaxation, and never engage to treat until one is procured. The supporter should be as uncomplicated

Ladies' Medical Guide, by S. Pancoast, MD, 1888

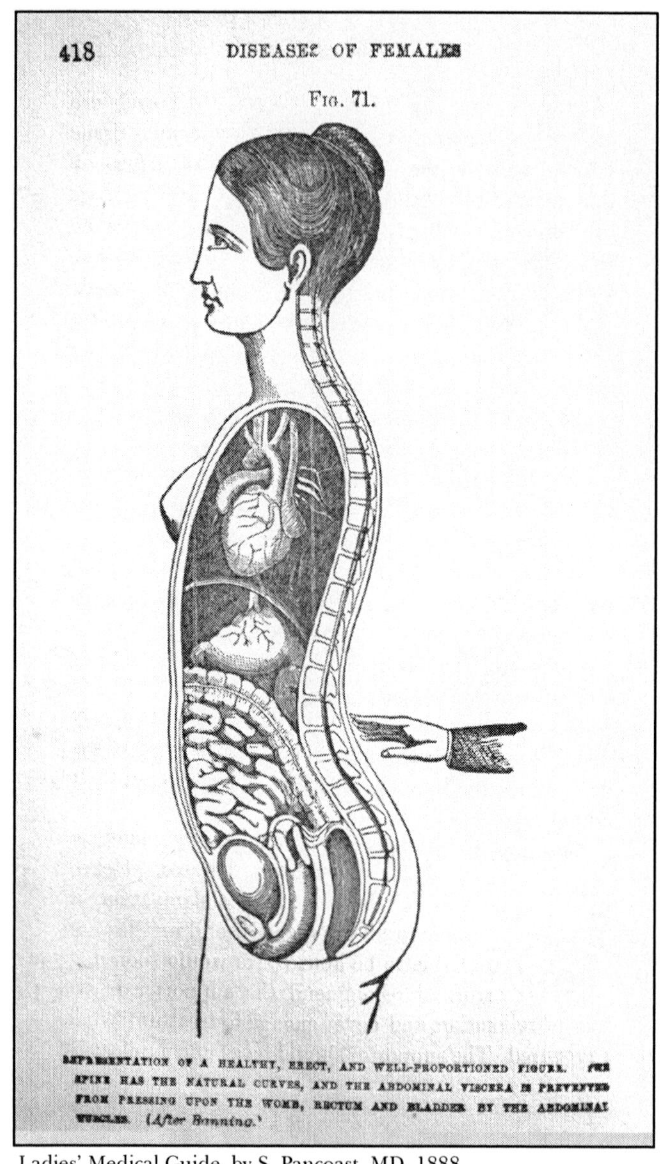

418 DISEASES OF FEMALES

FIG. 71.

REPRESENTATION OF A HEALTHY, ERECT, AND WELL-PROPORTIONED FIGURE. THE SPINE HAS THE NATURAL CURVES, AND THE ABDOMINAL VISCERA IS PREVENTED FROM PRESSING UPON THE WOMB, RECTUM AND BLADDER BY THE ABDOMINAL MUSCLES. (*After Banning.*)

Ladies' Medical Guide, by S. Pancoast, MD, 1888

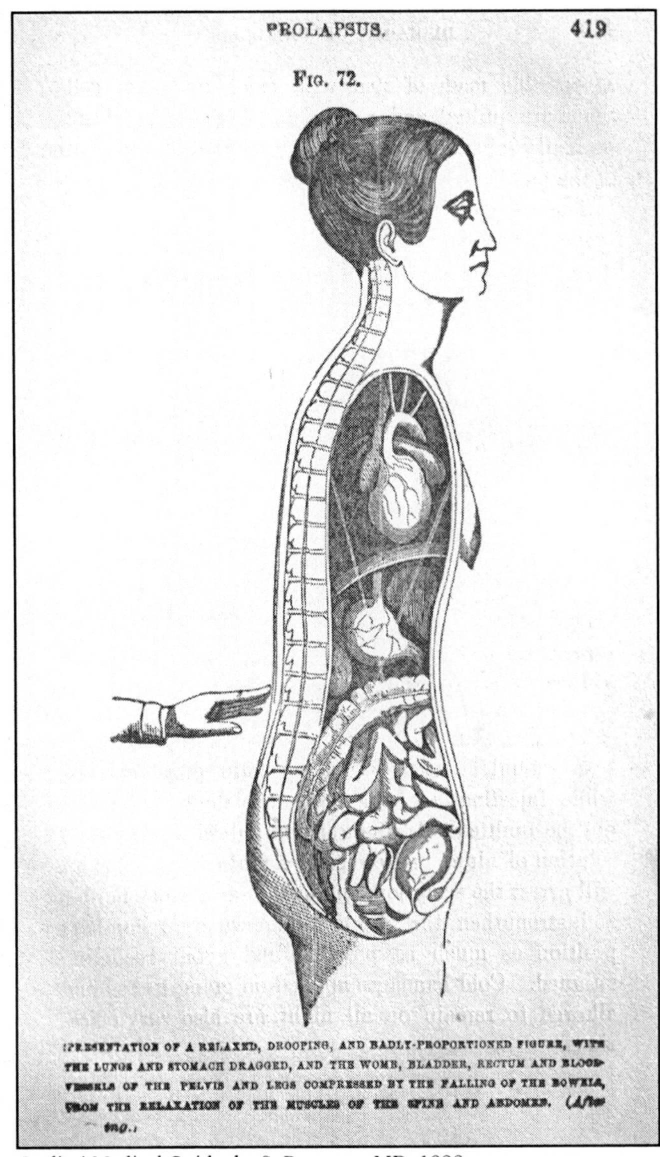

PROLAPSUS. 419

FIG. 72.

(REPRESENTATION OF A RELAXED, DROOPING, AND BADLY-PROPORTIONED FIGURE, WITH THE LUNGS AND STOMACH DRAGGED, AND THE WOMB, BLADDER, RECTUM AND BLOOD-VESSELS OF THE PELVIS AND LEGS COMPRESSED BY THE FALLING OF THE BOWELS, FROM THE RELAXATION OF THE MUSCLES OF THE SPINE AND ABDOMEN. (After [illegible]ing.)

Ladies' Medical Guide, by S. Pancoast, MD, 1888

420 DISEASES OF FEMALES.

as possible, made of steel with front and back pads Some are quilted and padded to such an extent as to be really injurious, by keeping up too great a warmth of the parts.

Tonics should be used to strengthen the general system. One of the following compounds may be used for this purpose:

℞ Sulphate cinchona,..........xxv grs.
Citrate iron, (soluable),......xxxv grs.

Make into twenty-four powders. Take one three times a day after each meal, in sweet wine.

℞ Precip. carbonate iron,..........ʒv.
Extract coniam,.........℈iv.
Balsam Peru,..................ʒj.
Simple syrup,..................℥viii.
Oil cinnamon,..................gtt. x.
Oil winter-green,..............gtt. x.
Pulv. gum Arabic,.............ʒij.

Mix.

Dose—two teaspoonsful three times a day, after meals To be well shaken before being used.

To give tone to the pelvic viscera, the cold hip bath should be used once a day, followed by friction while injections of cold water into the vagina must not be omitted. If there be any discharge, inject a solution of alum, one ounce to a pint of water. This will arrest the secretion, and at the same time harden and strengthen the vagina. Observe the recumbent position as much as possible, and avoid becoming fatigued. Cold bandages applied on going to bed and allowed to remain on all night, are also very efficacious.

Ladies' Medical Guide, by S. Pancoast, MD, 1888

The chief difficulty to overcome is the pressure around the waist by the use of corsets and wearing heavy skirts. Such pressure must be removed. The clothes should be loose and be suspended from the shoulders. Attention to this requirement cannot be too strongly impressed upon the mind of the patient.

The use of pessaries I utterly reprobate. They were used by the Egyptian, Greek, Roman and Arabian physicians, and are still recommended by some of the old-school practitioners of the present day. They are made of silver, gold, wood, cork, sponge and glass. Their use is merely palliative at best, while they often produce irritation and inflammation of the os-uteri and vagina, and, by consequence, lay the foundation of more formidable diseases, such as ulceration and cancer of the womb. The galvanic battery, in some cases, may be usefully employed, in connection with other treatment in prolapsus, especially if applied by or under the direction of an experienced practitioner.

b. RETROVERSION, OR RETROFLEXION OF UTERUS. —This is a displacement not so common as prolapsus. It may occur both in the pregnant and non-pregnant female. (*See Fig.* 73.) The uterus is here thrown back, the fundus resting against the rectum.

Symptoms.—If the retrocession is slight, there may be no well-marked symptoms. In other cases, the symptoms are dyspepsia and hysteria, and sometimes severe neuralgic pains in the breasts and along some portion of the spine; difficult breathing. Constipation is a common attendant; the uterus pressing against the rectum preventing the expulsion of the

36

Ladies' Medical Guide, by S. Pancoast, MD, 1888

In another such manual we find a similar treatise on "Prolapsus" from the beautifully illustrated and densely informative "Women's Guide to Health and Happiness" circa 1900.

This "Women's Guide" (author unknown) includes a similar recitation of prolapse symptoms, including the waxing and waning nature of prolapse: "Upon examination of the same displaced uterus, at different times of the day, it may be found to be more or less prolapsed, according to the condition of active exercise, or quiet, on which the parts may have been for some hours previous." Symptoms include urinary complaints,... frequent calls to urinate, dysuria (painful urination), or even retention of urine." The author(s) go on to recount these and other symptoms through which the diagnosis may be secured, reassuring that, "Should there be any doubt, however, the vaginal touch will verify the diagnosis." Causes include heavy lifting, heavy or tightly laced dresses, and getting up too soon after childbirth. Treatments include belladonna, distant derivatives of which are in use today for the treatment of overactive bladder, chamomile, an herbal remedy called china, and the homeopathic derivative nux vom. No surgery, no pessaries.

These ladies guides of the late 1800s were exhaustive references, including elaborate text on human anatomy replete with graphic illustrations, the basics of reproductive physiology and mating, the role to be played by refined ladies in the marital bed, the benefits of hygiene—the proper observance of which would "render... unnecessary.. seven-tenths of the calls received by physicians,"[1]—care of the eyes, children and the aged, and strict admonishments against "an evil which is hurl-

1 Ladies' Medical Guide by S. Pancoast, MD, 1888

DISEASES PECULIAR TO WOMEN. 249

near the time for the menstrual flow; and the discharge is so very acrid and corrosive that not only are the adjacent parts made sore, but the underclothing is made rotten and destroyed. *Dose:* Six globules.

The diet ought to be simple, but generally very nutritive. Coffee and tea ought to be avoided, and cocoa or arrowroot substituted. Regular exposure to the benign influence of the fresh air is commendable, but over-fatigue and prolonged standing should be sedulously avoided.

PROLAPSUS UTERI—FALLING OF THE WOMB.

This is one of the most common forms of uterine displacement. It occurs in three distinct, different degrees, to each of which some writers on the subject have affixed a different name. Thus, relaxation, or simple descent of the womb, is understood to indicate the first and least displacement downward, and to consist only in a simple bearing-down of the womb upon the upper portion of the vagina. In *prolapsus uteri*, the organ comes still lower down, and may present itself at the orifice of the vagina.

In *procerdentia uteri* there is actual protrusion of the organ, even the entire body of the womb being, in some cases, extended from the vulva. These are but different degrees of descent of the uterus in the line of the vagina. Upon examination of the same displaced uterus, at different times of the day, it may be found to be more or less prolapsed, according to the condition of active exercise, or quiet, in which the parts may have been for some hours previous.

Primary Symptoms.

The principal and primary symptoms of the descent of the womb are: dragging and aching pains in the small of the back, pulling and bearing-down pains in the lower part of the abdomen, sensation as if something would issue from the vagina; sufferings much worse from walking, or other exercise; the pains are often noticed to have come immediately after some exertion of an unusual kind, and after some

Women's Guide to Health and Happiness, circa 1900

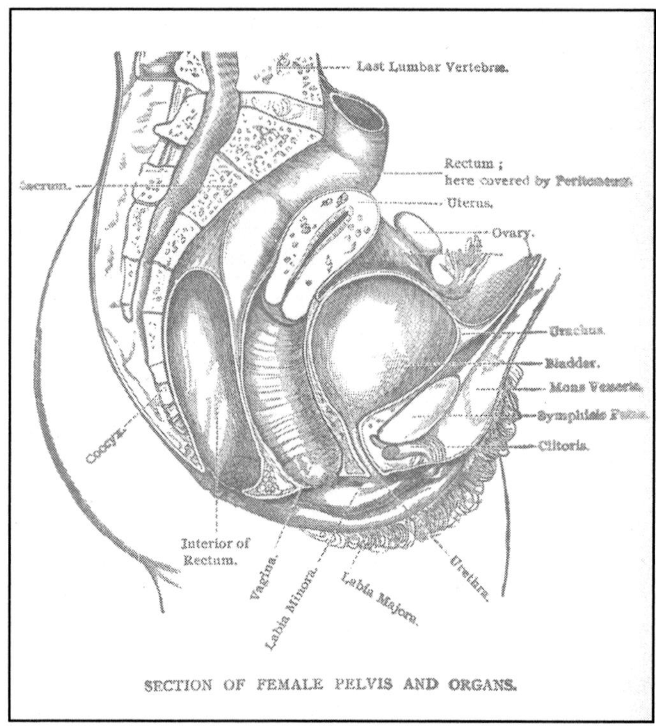

Women's Guide to Health and Happiness, circa 1900

250 DISEASES PECULIAR TO WOMEN.

more than ordinary muscular effort; frequent calls to urinate, dysuria (painful urination), or even retention of urine.

In the more fully developed forms of prolapsus, the history of the case, the attendant circumstances, and the external appearance of the mouth of the womb, and even of the entire body of the uterus itself, can hardly fail to render the diagnosis at once easy and certain. And if the falling of the womb is not so far developed as to give any such external signs, the severe aggravation from walking and from lifting, together with the relief experienced from lying down, render the case sufficiently clear. Should there be any doubt, however, the vaginal touch will verify the diagnosis.

Causes of the Falling of the Womb.

Prolapsus of the womb may arise from various causes, such as over-lifting or some other muscular exertion, or from an improper manner of dress, such as tight lacing, or the weight of heavy clothing dragging on the abdomen. In case of married women who have borne children, many cases of falling of the womb are caused by mismanagement.

Perhaps the bandage worn has been too tight, or has slipped up and the pressure has forced the bowels to press down upon the womb while in a relaxed condition, or, perhaps, the patient has gotten up from the bed too soon after confinement; the whole system being weak, it is very easy to do a little too much, and bring on injuries which are very often hard to relieve one's self of. In cases of displacement of the womb, the recumbent posture is a necessary requirement, together with the properly selected remedy; a cure can very frequently be obtained.

Treatment.

Belladonna. Pressure, as though all the contents of the abdomen would issue through the genital organs. This is particularly felt early in the morning; sensation of heat and dryness in the vagina. Pains in the pelvic region, which come on suddenly and cease suddenly, or

Women's Guide to Health and Happiness, circa 1900

DISEASES PECULIAR TO WOMEN. 251

feeling in the back as if it would break, hindering motion, suppression of the stool and of urine.

Chamomilla. Frequent pressure toward the uterus, like labor pains, with frequent desire to urinate, often passing large quantities of colorless urine. Frequent discharge of clotted blood, with tearing pain in the veins of the legs, and violent labor-like pains in the uterus. Contrary to her condition in health, she is always out of humor, particularly at her menstrual periods, when she is headstrong, even unto quarreling. She can hardly speak a pleasant word, and has to restrain herself in order to do so.

China. In cases where the prolapsus and attendant symptoms were superinduced by losses of fluids, particularly of blood. She has much ringing in the ears, a sense of distention in the abdomen, which is not relieved by eructations.

Nux Vom. Prolapsus uteri, from straining by lifting. Pressure toward the genital organs, early in the morning, in bed, or during a walk, with a sensation of drawing in the abdomen. Constipation of large, hard, difficult stools, or small stools, with frequent urging. Pain in the small of the back, preventing her from turning over in bed. Frequent urination; she passes little, and often, with much burning pain. The prolapsus of long standing is often accompanied with dry cough, and a sense of constriction around the lower part of the abdomen.

THE CHANGE OF LIFE—MENOPAUSE.

After a certain number of years, woman lays aside those functions with which she has been endowed for the perpetuation of the species, and resumes once more that exclusively individual life which had been her's when a child. The evening of her days approaches, and if she has observed the precepts of wisdom, she may look forward to a long and placid period of rest, blessed with health, honored, yes, loved with a purer flame than any which she inspired in the bloom of youth and beauty.

But ere this haven of rest is reached, there is a crisis to pass, which

Women's Guide to Health and Happiness, circa 1900

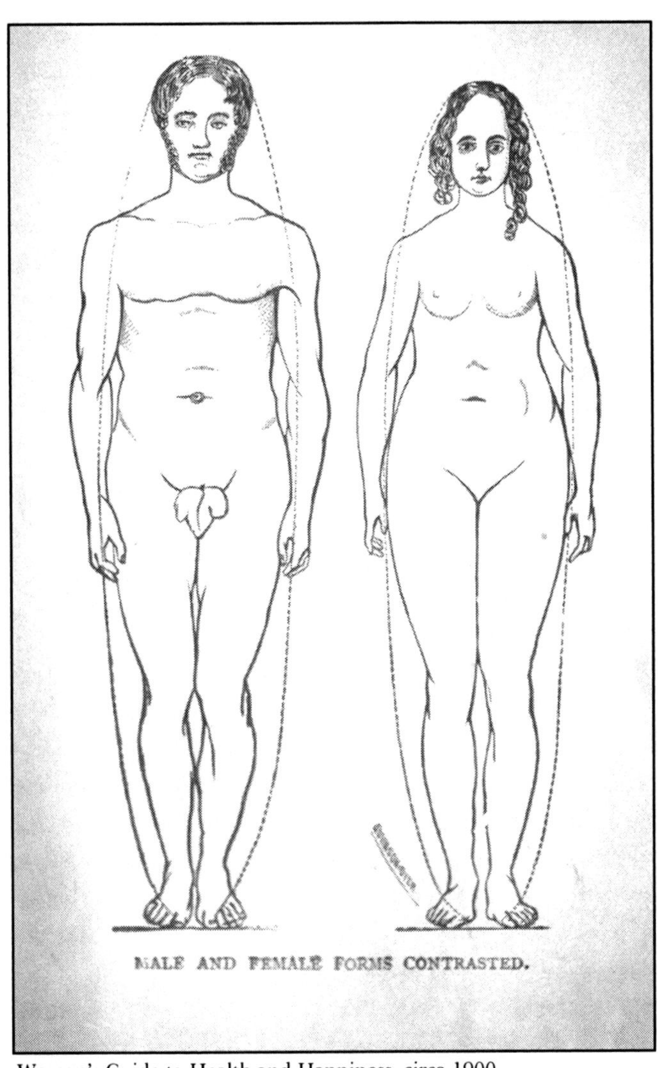

Women's Guide to Health and Happiness, circa 1900

ing thousands on thousands every year to a loathsome and untimely grave—an evil threatening the utter extinction of the human race!... The truly conscientious physician cannot shirk his responsibility to the public, but should lift up his voice in earnest... against the horrible vice... of Onanism or Masturbation, or in still plainer terms, Self-Pollution!"[2] This section on the horrors of self-abuse, titled "Startling Facts in Plain Words," goes on for 27 terrifying pages, followed by chapters on care of the newborn and nice ways for ladies to style their hair to reflect modesty and impeccable breeding. All this and prolapse too!

Today, nonsurgical prolapse therapies include pessary, Colpexin™ device, Fembrace™, and the largely unproven prolapse-treatment potential of Kegel exercises. Yes, that's right, contrary to popular belief we have no medical data or anecdotal clinical experience to reassure us that Kegels cure prolapse.

Pessaries

Prosthetic support gadgets for vaginal prolapse are called pessaries They come in a variety of shapes and sizes made of latex, plastic or silicone. Pessaries are an ancient therapy, the earliest being smooth stones and root vegetables, such as potatoes. Don't ask. The best pessary is one that the patient can insert and remove herself, fits with no discomfort, and holds the prolapse in place without fail during all levels of activity.

Patients are rarely neutral about pessaries, being either thoroughly mortified at the mere suggestion of wearing the vaginal equivalent of a whiplash collar, or as enthusiastic as a fashionista (and you know who you are!)

2 Women's Guide to Health and Happiness, circa 1900

The Modern Prolapse Pessary

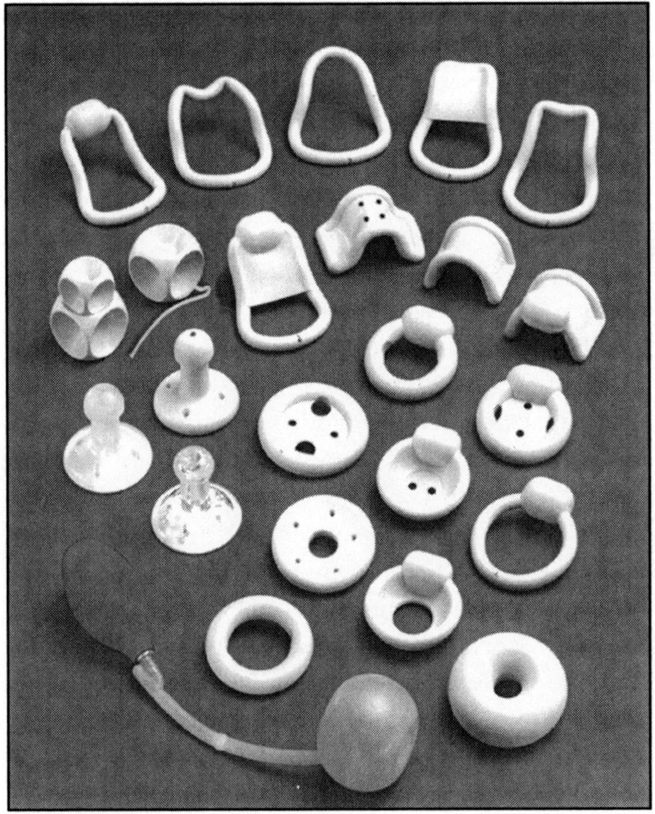

With permission from Cooper Surgical (www.coopersurgical.com)

at a Barneys sale at the prospect of avoiding a trip to the operating room. Pessaries are fantastic for women with prolapse who are in between babies, women who want surgery but can't arrange the time off that they'll need to recuperate, women who can't have surgery because of poor health, or women who just don't want an operation unless there is no other choice. I've had patients walk in ready to sign up for surgery, walk out with a "temporary" pessary and vanish for years because the pessary was so easy to use. Many of these pessary converts return eventually for a new replacement pessary or to "finally get that surgery done." Pessaries today look like space station furnishings for Astronaut Barbie.

Be not afraid, your gynecologist can help you find a pessary that works for you. My personal favorite is the ring plate pessary (in the middle, two large and two small holes) because it is the easiest for the patient to insert and remove, particularly for women who have used diaphragms in the past; the shape, insertion and removal techniques are exactly the same as a diaphragm. But the ring pessary rests on the levator ani/Kegel muscles, so if the muscles are thin and weak, this pessary will be difficult or impossible to retain, slipping out with coughing, bending, lifting or defecating. In such cases I move on either to the Gelhorn for uterine prolapse (the trio of stemmed pessaries, on the left) or the Gehrung for severe cystocele (the bridge shaped pessaries, with and without bolster, upper right corner). Neither the Gelhorn nor the Gehrung need strong levator muscles to rest on, and that's good, but both are more difficult for the patient to learn to insert and remove, and that can be bad for patients with an active sex life. Other pessaries come with bolsters along the rim (to the right of the simple ring plate, with various bolsters on the rim) designed to reduce urine leakage in women with the common combination of urinary leakage and prolapse. The balloon-style pessary with long stem (bottom) can be inflated and deflated, a bit easier than inserting and removing a potato. To reiterate, pessaries don't cure prolapse, but they can provide a very effective short- or long-term treatment. They are ideal for women who are in between pregnancies, or who cannot or prefer not to undergo surgery.

Whether or not pessary use slows the progress of prolapse is not known, although I, along with many clinicians, believe that it probably does. In fact on a few occasions I have seen women "shrink-wrap" around forgotten pessaries, some left in for years at a time, and upon extraction, the prolapse is effectively gone because the scarring and stricture caused by the neglected pessary holds the uterus, bladder and rectum in place, but this is very uncommon.

Most pessary users must be refitted within five years. Pessaries should be replaced if they are cracked, pitted or have a foul odor after cleaning. Pessaries are cleaned with bath soap and towel dried. They should not be boiled or soaked in antiseptic solutions.

The newest, and possibly the most clever, pessary looks like a lollipop on a string, its simple design belying its overlapping benefits. The Colpexin™ device is designed to remodel vaginal laxities while passively exercising the levator ani muscles as you go about your daily business. Colpexin™ is available throughout Europe as an over-the-counter pelvic device, available in one size only. Here, in the United States, you must see a physician or other qualified clinician for a fitting, since there are five different sizes to match your personal anatomy. Colpexin™ is the only prolapse gadget with bona fide medical research data showing that it reduces mild to moderate prolapse in addition to increasing pelvic muscle fitness. During the clinical trial, participating women wore their Colpexin™ for 16 weeks, during which time it toned and stimulated the levator ani muscles. At the end of the 16-week preclinical trial, 81% of the women had measurably lesser prolapse on examination by the doctor, 63% had stronger, more fit levator muscles, and 92-100% were happy with their results, reporting better vaginal muscle fitness and bladder control, stating they would recommend Colpexin™ to a friend. Colpexin™ is ideal for women with less than severe prolapse and/or weak Kegel muscles. Why stop at 16 weeks? If you have a vagina, Kegels are your best friend south of the bellybutton, and with Colpexin™ this exercise is on autopilot.

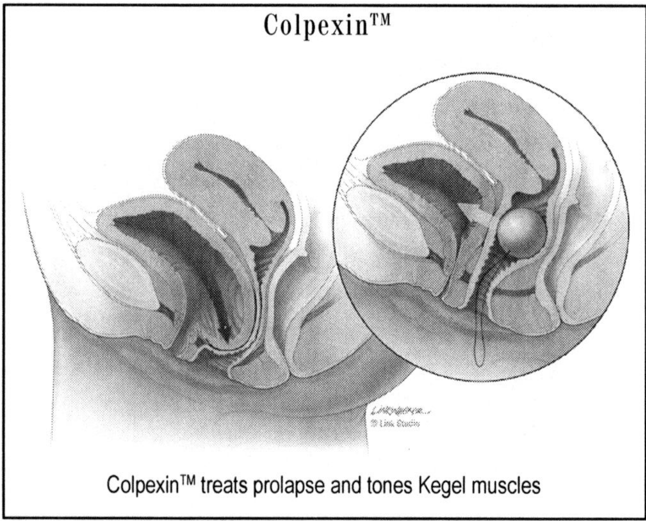

Colpexin™ treats prolapse and tones Kegel muscles

With permission from Adamed, Inc. (www.colpexin.com)

Garments

The Fembrace™ is a girdle style undergarment designed to hold pelvic prolapse in place from the outside, similar in concept to the medical truss used to hold an inguinal hernia in place. While there is no medical research or clinical trials using this device, testimonials on file with the company confirm its comfort and utility. The brace is marketed as:

> *"A revolutionary new support garment for relief of the painful symptoms of Genital Prolapse (Prolapsed Uterus, Cystocele, Rectocele, Enterocele) and Varicose Veins of the Vulva (Vulvar Varicosities). The V-Brace™ provides the same support as placing your hand on the vaginal area and applying pressure upwards. The V-Brace™ provides this support more effectively and consistently without slipping or chafing."*

On the market since 2000, the brace was designed by surgical supply retailers and is available without a doctor's prescription. It may not be the sexiest tool in the shed, but I've had women stuffing rolled up pads into stiff girdles as a homemade strategy for severe prolapse since I started in this business. These "stuffing the jockstrap" prolapse sufferers are well served by the more user-friendly alternative of the Fembrace™, which is ideal for women who cannot or choose not to use a pessary or to undergo reconstructive surgery.

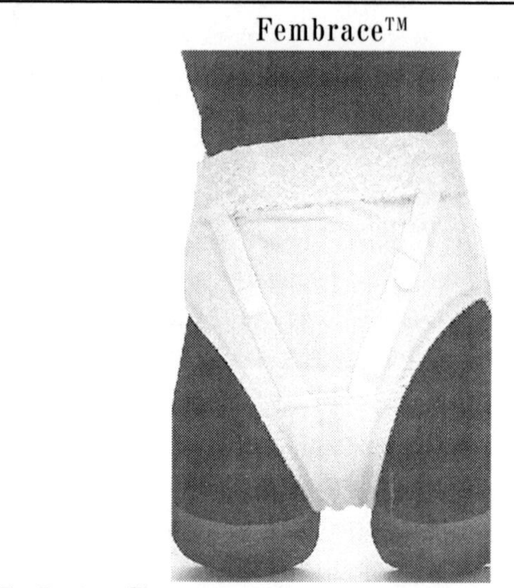

The Fembrace™ is a garment designed to support severe pelvic prolapse from outside of the body and is available without a prescription

With permission from Fembrace, Inc. (www.fembrace.com)

Kegel Exercise

Kegels are the dental floss of the female pelvis. If you have a vagina and you're old enough to vote, then you should be Kegeling every day.

What are the benefits of levator muscle fitness? There is plenty of data showing that Kegels are good for bladder control and a few studies that show Kegels will give you a stronger orgasm, but none shedding light on whether or not Kegels will hold your vaginal parts in place, nor even how best to do Kegels.

In the world of medical research, if you want to know the latest on Kegel exercise, there is no single clinical scientist today more devoted to pelvic muscle fitness than Dr. Kari Bo, Professor in the Department of Sports Medicine, Norwegian School of Sports Sciences, in Oslo, Norway. Her efforts are a clear extension of the original concept put forward by Dr. Arnold Kegel himself, including many papers on the use of Kegel exercise to improve pelvic muscle fitness and reduce urinary incontinence. In a recent review Dr. Bo combed the medical literature to see whether there was any data showing that Kegel exercises treat or cure prolapse. Finding only one small study addressing this issue, Dr. Bo concludes, "There is an urgent need for more...trials with high methodological quality, use of valid and reproducible methods to assess degree of prolapse, and appropriate training protocols to evaluate the effect of pelvic floor muscle therapy in the prevention and treatment of pelvic organ prolapse."[3]

When it comes to Kegels and prolapse one can only apply a healthy dose of common sense; it is probably very helpful to keep your levator ani muscles in good shape

3 Bo K. Can pelvic floor muscle training prevent and treat pelvic organ prolapse? Acta Obstet Gynecol Scand 2006.

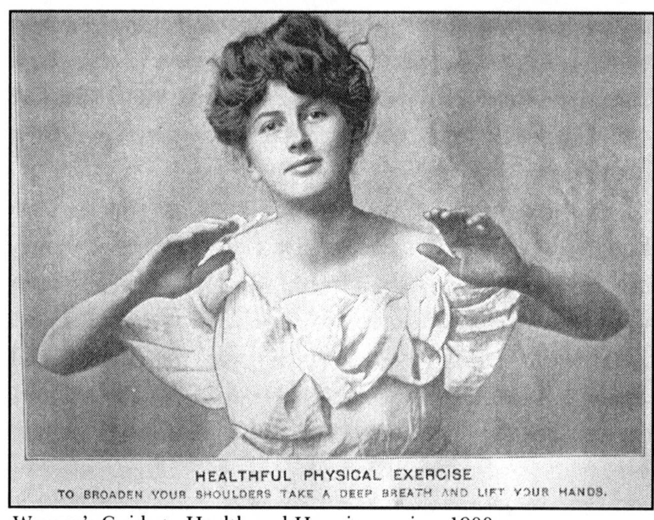

HEALTHFUL PHYSICAL EXERCISE
TO BROADEN YOUR SHOULDERS TAKE A DEEP BREATH AND LIFT YOUR HANDS.
Women's Guide to Health and Happiness, circa 1900

with Kegel exercises and, as recommended by Dr. Bo, making a habit of "conscious contraction during increase in abdominal pressure in daily activities." If you have moderate prolapse, Kegels might reduce the severity of the bulge or arrest the slow increase in laxity that most prolapse patients experience over the years, but the science behind that assumption is simply not available. Other than the single study looking at Kegel exercise and prolapse after using the Colpexin™ device, no data is available on whether or not Kegel exercise prevents or treats pelvic organ prolapse.

In my experience, Kegels can help a woman with prolapse by improving muscle bulk which makes pessary fitting easier, because a woman with fit levators can usually be fitted for the more user-friendly ring pessary. Women with thin, skinny levator muscles usually cannot retain the ring, and must be fitted for pessaries that are more difficult, or even impossible, for the patient to insert and remove herself, requiring regular visits for pessary care and making sexual intercourse very tricky. On the other hand, if you have severe prolapse, it is very unlikely that Kegels will do much to pull your parts back into position, any more than you could expect sit-ups to cure a large groin or bellybutton hernia.

So if you want to make sure you Kegel correctly ask for a pelvic muscle check at your next gynecologic checkup.[4] Below is a quick, 5 second test of coordination, strength and endurance of this muscle group that your doctor can use to score your "Kegel Score" at your next visit.[5]

4 See Appendix.

5 Romanzi et al simple test of pelvic muscle contraction during pelvic examination; correlation to surface electromyography. Neurourol Urodyn 1999.

5 Second Kegel Score Test				
	0	**1**	**2**	**3**
Pressure	None	Weak	Moderate	Strong
Duration	None	<1 Second	1-5 Seconds	>5 Seconds
Displacement	None	Slight Rotation	Full Rotation	Gripped

Your Score: ________/9

Pressure generated around the examining fingers is rated for duration of maximal contraction effort and the degree to which the muscle contraction rotates the fingers toward the pubic bone. For scores of 0-3, I strongly recommend referral to a pelvic floor physical therapy clinician for at least four sessions of monitored pelvic floor work with adjunctive electrical stimulation. If you're that weak you need professional help whether you have pelvic symptoms or not. There is no way you will be able to do it on your own; you need a coach. For scores of 7-9, I recommend daily Kegels to maintain your excellent levator muscle coordination, endurance and strength, doing 2-3 sets of 10 contractions, each held for a count of 5-10 (as able) daily along with 30-50 "quick flick" contractions intermixed with your sustained contractions. Women with 7-9 scores will be able to do this without the coaching provided by pelvic floor physical therapy. For women in the intervening score range of 4-6, I recommend a pelvic floor clinician for monitored work if you have pelvic symptoms, and work on your own using the 7-9 score regimen if you are symptom free.

If you can't talk your doctor into "scoring your levators," use your man. If he can't feel a thing, you need pelvic floor physical therapy. If he seems impressed, you're on the right track. If he looks a little scared, you're Kegeling like a pro.

So, short of surgery, you have all sorts of options. Pessaries that hold in prolapse, pessaries that hold in prolapse and reduce urinary leakage, pessaries that hold in prolapse and Kegel exercise you all day long, or groovy girdles, any and all of which can be augmented by Kegels à la cart, or my personal favorite, Kegels "à la man."

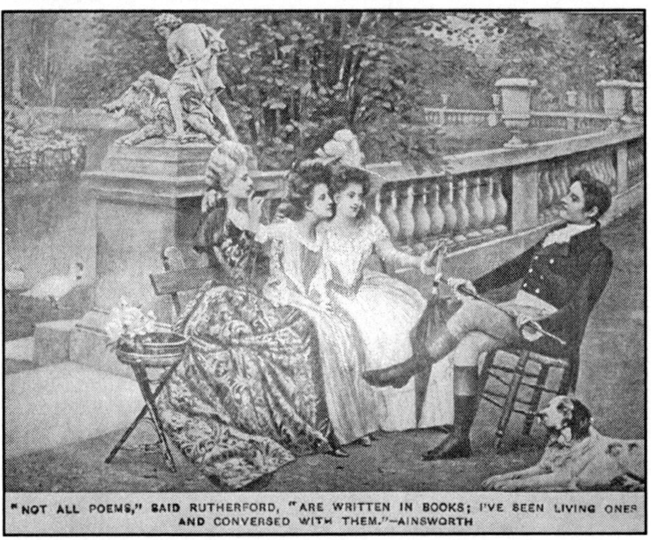

"NOT ALL POEMS," SAID RUTHERFORD, "ARE WRITTEN IN BOOKS; I'VE SEEN LIVING ONES AND CONVERSED WITH THEM."—AINSWORTH

Women's Guide to Health and Happiness, circa 1900

THREE

Renovations

So you tried all the pessaries and they just don't fit, or won't stay in, or it presses on the bladder or it presses on the rectum, or it's just not your thing. If that's you, then it's time for the operating room. Prolapse can give you bladder problems, bowel symptoms, pain and disability, and can interfere with your body-image something fierce. Just like hernia or knee surgery, female reconstructive pelvic surgery focuses on restoring support, function and normal contour to a body part that is broken, bulging and not working right. As with all reconstructive surgeries, it is possible that the problem may come back after surgical repair. Most prolapse repairs last a very long time, some last a lifetime, and some need tweaking after a relatively short time.

The risk of recurrence after prolapse reconstructive surgery is no different in the pelvis than in any other area of the body. We all know someone who's gone back to redo a knee repair, or signs up for second facelift, or tears the shoulder again after rotator cuff repair, or has more than one spinal operation for a slipped disc, or sprouts another hernia after the first operation. So understand that while most prolapse operations last a long time, and many a lifetime, pelvic prolapse might come back down after reconstructive surgery due to circumstances beyond the control of you or your surgeon. The most recent data on durability of prolapse surgery showed a 17% reoperation rate 10 years after initial reconstructive operation, reinforcing the impetus for ongoing collaboration to improve the durability and further reduce recurrence of pelvic organ prolapse repair. A durable, potentially lifelong repair is one that fixes all defects whether they bother you or not, includes the judicious consideration of graft material, and takes a careful look at bladder function before surgery, not afterwards.

The recommendation to include hysterectomy in prolapse repair is deeply ingrained in the guiding principles of American gynecology. Three (mis)guiding principles underpin this entrenched clinical bias. Let's take a look.

The Holy Trinity of Hysterectomy

Unlike most other reconstructive operations, pelvic prolapse surgery involves organs that might turn malignant as a woman ages, highlighting the first argument in favor of the unwritten rule that prolapse surgery should include hysterectomy (removal of the uterus) and/or oophorectomy (removal of the ovaries).

Traditional gynecologic training teaches young doctors that the uterus is only for childbearing and that the uterus and ovaries should be removed at the time of any gynecologic surgery in women over age 45, since the woman is unlikely to bear more children and removal of the uterus and ovaries will prevent cancer. The average woman has a 2-3% lifetime risk of uterine or ovarian cancer, both of which peak in incidence around age 60. With no reliable screening test for ovarian cancer, it is obvious why gynecologic tradition favors hysterectomy and removal of ovaries in women close to or already in menopause (average age 51), when the ovaries stop producing eggs and estrogen. If the ovaries "aren't doing anything" why not remove them and reduce the woman's cancer risks? Ovarian cancer is an aggressive, difficult to diagnose, deadly disease, similar to melanoma and pancreatic cancer. By the time you have symptoms, ovarian cancer is typically in an advanced stage and survival rates are very low. Women with increased risks for gynecologic cancer (personal history of breast cancer, strong family history of colon, breast or ovarian cancer, BRCA gene-positive women, exposure to high dose radiation or DES) have up to a 50% risk of gynecologic cancer and often welcome the opportunity to take care of two health concerns at once by including hysterectomy and/or oophorectomy (removal of the ovaries) along with their prolapse repair. Whether average or high risk, this cancer concern is the most relevant of pro-hysterectomy arguments and deserves thoughtful consideration by any woman undergoing prolapse surgery.

On the other side of this cancer-prevention argument, I always ask the same question: "If you did not have any prolapse, would your gynecologist have any good reason to chase you down the street, frantically insisting that you remove your uterus or ovaries?" If the answer is no, and you are willing to go on living with your average ovar-

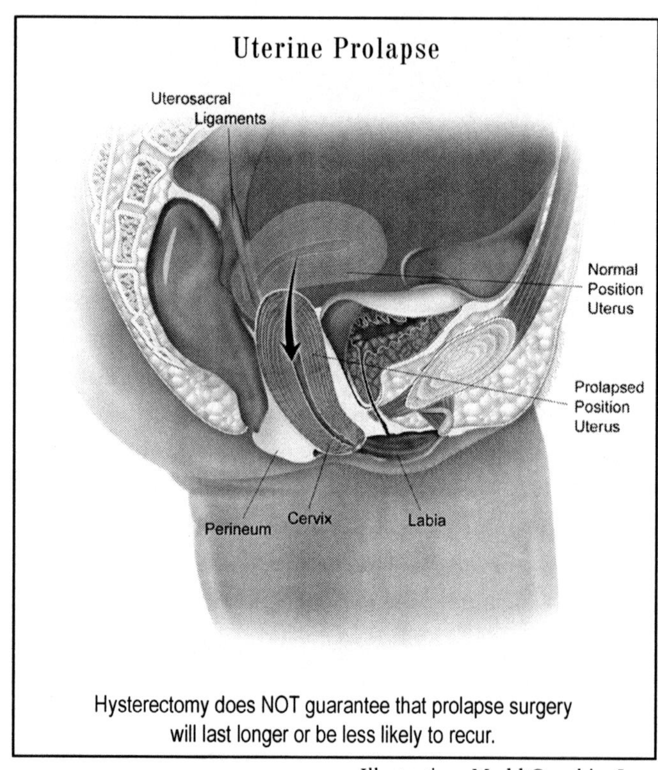

Illustration: Madd Graphix, Inc.

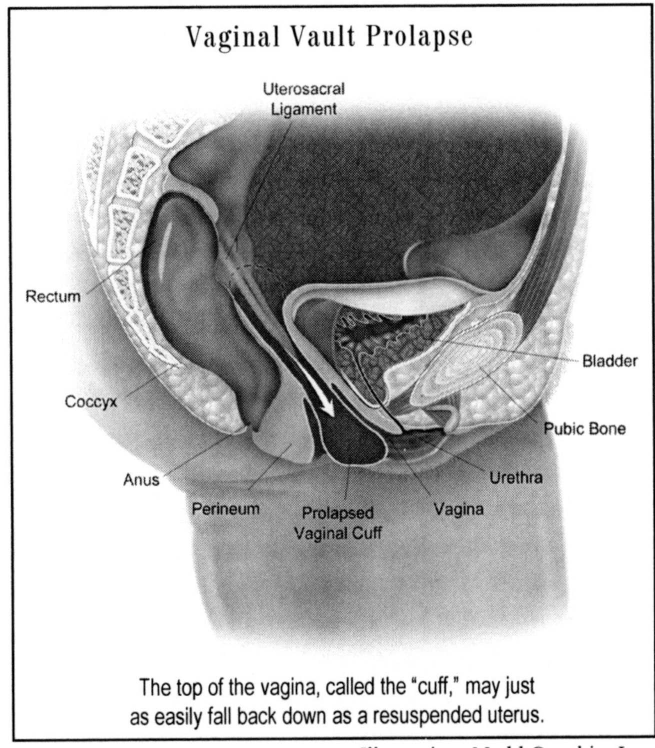

The top of the vagina, called the "cuff," may just as easily fall back down as a resuspended uterus.

Illustration: Madd Graphix, Inc.

ian and uterine cancer risks, you are an ideal candidate for uterine resuspension prolapse repair, which leaves all organs in place while fixing the prolapse just as well as, if not better than, prolapse repair done with hysterectomy.

Which introduces the second traditional justification for hysterectomy at the time of prolapse repair: "The uterus will fall back down again if we don't take it out." This argument is as flimsy as the cancer-prevention argument is worthy. The uterus is not a weight or a tractor-pull contest. The uterus is held in place at the top of the vagina by the sturdy uterosacral ligaments. The uterus does not fall down because it is heavy, it prolapses because the ligaments give way. Repair of the ligaments is crucial to successful uterine prolapse surgery; if the ligaments are not taken care of, the surgeon will simply turn the uterine prolapse into a vaginal prolapse.

The uterosacral ligaments soften during pregnancy and can stretch during childbirth, making uterine prolapse a childbirth injury in most cases, even though the actual prolapse may not appear until 20 or 30 years later. The nonpregnant uterus is not a weight and it will not stretch the ligaments out again after surgery. Fix the ligaments and you fix the prolapse.

Hysterectomy does NOT guarantee that prolapse surgery will last longer or be less likely to recur. The top of the vagina, called the "cuff," may just as easily fall back down as a resuspended uterus.

The final argument for removing the uterus at time of hysterectomy is that "hysterectomy won't hurt/might even help your sex life." Many women cringe at this incredulous advice, but believe it or not, there actually are studies showing that hysterectomy has no effect or even improves sexual function. However, if you read between the lines, you often find that this "benefit" is probably due to the amelioration of the symptoms that have previously had a negative effect on sexual function,"[1] while other researchers caution us that "There are reasons to believe that removal of the uterus can have adverse effects on female sexual functioning by disrupting the anatomical relations in the pelvis. ...A critical attitude towards the indications of hysterectomy remains mandatory."[2] If you have enormous and painful fibroids in your uterus, or your female organs are glued together and chronically inflamed from endometriosis, the uterus may well be extremely painful during sexual intercourse, and women in these situations will report far less pain and far greater pleasure during sex after a hysterectomy. But many hysterectomies are done in women where the uterus is not painful or disabling.

So what happens if a woman has a uterus removed that is not in and of itself a source of pain or discomfort? One very troubling study showed a serious impact on sexuality in women ages 39-45 who underwent hysterectomy for irregular bleeding as compared to women with the same abnormal bleeding who underwent a uterine-sparing treatment called endometrial ablation instead of hysterectomy. Between 70-82% of the hysterectomy patients reported extreme negative impact on sexual arousal, libido and vaginal lubrication. Other research shows that hysterectomy reduces blood flow to the vagina and ovaries and this reduction in blood flow correlates with a drop in sex hormone levels in the bloodstream. Decreased blood flow to the vagina may also diminish capillary blood flow

---

1 Mokate T, et al Hysterectomy and sexual function J Br Menop Soc 2006.

2 Maas CP et al The effect of hysterectomy on sexual functioning Annu Rev Sex Res 2003.

in the genital skin, sexual engorgement and sexual pleasure. Sweet Mother of God, the uterus is an integral body part and not a Lego™ piece! Who knew?

This holy trinity of hysterectomy advocacy is, in each and every facet, open to challenge. (1) Hysterectomy may well have a negative impact on your sex life unless your uterus is a source of pain or sexual dysfunction all by itself, (2) the prolapse repair holds up just as well whether you leave the uterus in or take it out, and (3) gynecologic cancer risk in the average woman is quite low. It is very reasonable to decide to leave the uterus and ovaries in at time of prolapse surgery unless there is good and specific gynecologic reason to take them out. Prolapse alone is simply not one of those reasons.

And remember the argument that the ovaries are "doing nothing" after menopause and are therefore no more than potential sites of future cancer?

Compelling new data shows that the menopausal ovary may well lengthen your life.

A recent epidemiologic study showed that removing ovaries before age 70 has a negative impact on life expectancy; in other words, for reasons we do not yet understand, removing the ovaries before that age appears to shorten a woman's life.[3] This controversial and fascinating study will surely beget more research that will confirm or refute the original work. In the meantime, beware the mighty menopausal ovary; it may do you more good than harm.

3 Parker et al Ovarian conservation at the time of hysterectomy for benign disease Obstet Gynecol 2005.

"As I have aged, I have become fonder of my ovaries and am less likely to prophylactically remove mine or those of others." Rebecca G. Rogers, MD[1]

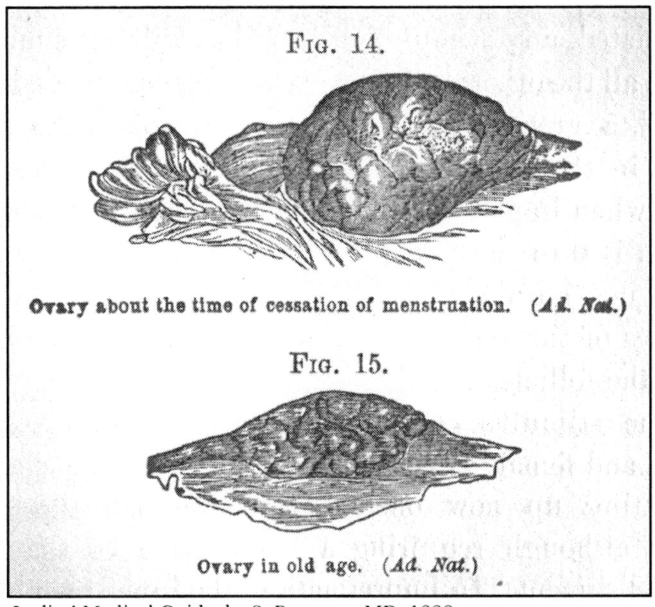

Ladies' Medical Guide, by S. Pancoast, MD, 1888

1 Rogers RG. Castration at the time of benign hysterectomy, The Female Patient 2008.

Uterine Resuspension

Now that you have the tools to decide whether or not your uterus will be removed as part of your prolapse repair, let's go over the different uterine prolapse surgery options.

Except for one operation called the Manchester procedure, operations to fix uterine prolapse were all originally designed to begin with hysterectomy followed by resuspension of the top of the vagina in the area where the cervix used to be, called the "vaginal cuff". The original uterine resuspension operation, the Manchester procedure, was first described in 1888. The Manchester uses the bottommost edge of the uterosacral ligament complex, called the cardinal ligament to elevate a prolapsed uterus. The other uterine suspensions all appeared on the gynecologic scene over the last 15 years, each of which is a modification of a hysterectomy-based vaginal cuff suspension, based on one of three anatomic approaches: suspension to the sacrospinous ligament, suspension to the sacrum bone, or suspension to the uterosacral ligaments. These uterine-sparing procedures are labeled *uterine resuspension*, or the synonymous *hysteropexy*.

The two things patients need to know with any reconstructive operation are:

1. How long will it last?
2. What are the most common complications?

Let's review the options for uterine prolapse repair.

#1: Cardinal Ligament; the Manchester Procedure

The Manchester-Fothergill procedure is the grandmother of all uterine suspension prolapse repairs. This handy vaginal procedure was, until the mid-1990s, the only available operation to correct uterine prolapse without resorting to hysterectomy. As a result of decades of hysterectomy-focused prolapse repair dogma, you will be hard-pressed to find the few surgeons who offer this operation. The Manchester-Fothergill procedure was first introduced in 1888, devised to resuspend the uterus in young women toiling in the sheepshearing industry. Repetitive lifting of sheep caused the uterus to drop in some women, making childbearing difficult. You can't have a baby without a uterus, and it's fairly difficult to get pregnant if your cervix is hanging out of your body, and so this procedure was originally devised to reposition the uterus inside the vagina, preserving fertility. The Manchester procedure is done through the vagina. To lift the uterus, the vaginal edge of the uterosacral ligament complex, a less robust portion called the "cardinal" ligaments, are repositioned to wrap in front of the cervix, at which point the cervix is shortened so that it cannot be seen or felt at the vaginal opening.

When to Tinker with the Cervix

This mandatory shortening of the cervix is unique to the Manchester uterine resuspension. With other suspensions, cervical shortening is done on a case-by-case basis. A normal cervical length is around two inches, or about four cm. Some are longer, some shorter, and in the course of a woman's life the shape, bulkiness and length of the cervix varies. For reasons that we do not understand the cervix can elongate impressively when the uterus prolapses, just like Pinocchio's nose. Cervical elongation, also called "cervical hypertrophy," rarely occurs in any other setting, and we do not know why prolapse predisposes the cervix to this bizarre transformation. It is not common, in my experience, occurring in about 10% of my prolapse patients.

When I say elongated cervix, I mean loooong. Some look like elephant trunks, reaching lengths of 10 cm or more, double or triple the length of the uterus above it, sticking out of the vagina even when the prolapsed uterus is replaced into normal position. Acting like a battering ram, an elongated cervix will push out any pessary you might try, making surgery the only treatment option.

A hypertrophied cervix must be shortened at time of prolapse repair, otherwise it juts into and fills up the vagina after uterine resuspension like a stalactite hanging from the roof of a limestone cave. Being that cervical hypertrophy doesn't happen all that often, most uterine resuspensions may be done without any tailoring of cervical structure whatsoever, but with the Manchester cervical shortening is always done, whether there is cervical elongation or not.

Shortening a normal-length cervix always struck me as unnecessary. I never could figure out, nor did my mentors have the answer, why it was originally designed to always be done during a Manchester procedure even in women with normal-sized cervices. Were all the cervices of these young nineteenth-century sheepshearers hypertrophied? Or was the cervix shortened to reduce the likelihood that it would project outside the vagina in the event that the prolapse recurred? We may never know. If your cervix is extremely long, it can and should be shortened at the time of your prolapse repair. If your cervix is of normal length and you are scheduled for a Manchester procedure, talk to your surgeon about the possibility of leaving the cervical shortening portion of the operation out.

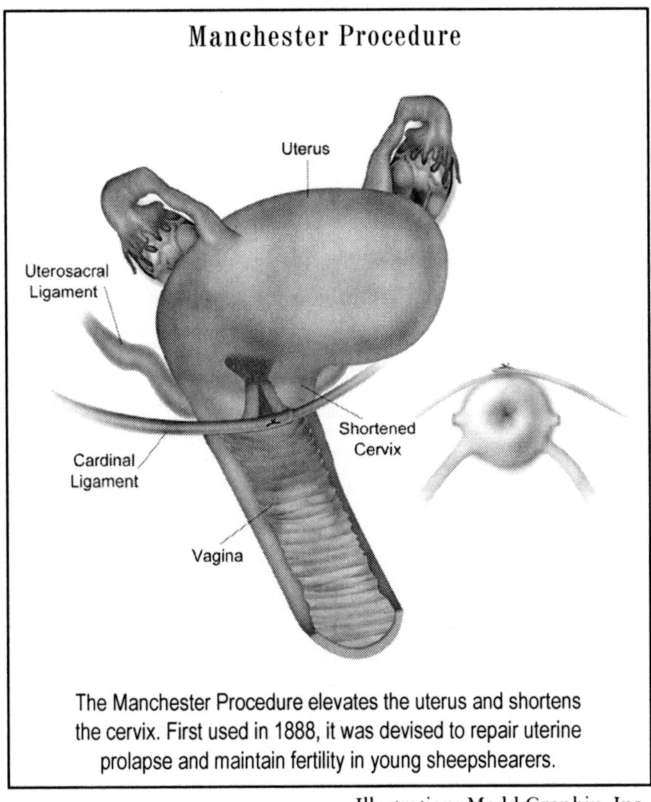

The Manchester Procedure elevates the uterus and shortens the cervix. First used in 1888, it was devised to repair uterine prolapse and maintain fertility in young sheepshearers.

Illustration: Madd Graphix, Inc.

Research data from my colleagues at nearby Mt. Sinai Hospital here in New York City showed that the Manchester takes much less time to perform, with less blood loss, minimal complications on the operating table and a quicker recuperation as compared to vaginal hysterectomy done for uterine prolapse repair. For advanced elderly patients with severe prolapse who cannot use a pessary but are poor surgical risks due to illness, the Manchester is an excellent option. We owe a lot to the Manchester. Until recently, it was the only procedure designed to correct uterine prolapse without taking the uterus out.

So what are the possible complications of the Manchester? The most common is burial of the cervix beneath the vaginal skin if the skin heals in a way that completely covers the center of the shortened cervix. Turkish colleagues recently published the only study reporting any complication data on the Manchester, finding a 12% incidence of cervical scarring beneath the vaginal skin. Should this occur, it is easily remedied with a minor revision to open the cervix again.

How long does it last? We don't really know. Despite the fact that the Manchester suspension has been in use since 1888, the same Turkish study is only one reporting how well the Manchester operation holds up over time. This durability data showed a 4% recurrence of uterine prolapse in women who had undergone Manchester three years earlier, meaning that 96% of these women's repairs were holding up well after three years. My personal experience over the past 15 years shows that no matter how long it lasts, the Manchester procedure does not do a great job of replacing the uterus all the way up at the very top of the vagina, typically pulling the uterus back up about midway, and doing little to address laxity in the remainder of the untouched uterosacral ligament complex. Whether this cardinal ligament suspension is the best option in all cases of uterine prolapse has yet to be determined.

The Manchester is the least invasive of all the uterine suspensions, done vaginally without entry into the pelvic cavity or deep tissue layers around the vagina, or use of the bony ligaments of the pelvis.

Up until the first half of the twentieth century there was no such thing as surgery to prevent disease, only surgery as a last resort to save someone who would surely die if nothing was done (severe infections, cancer, farming accidents, and the like). Safe and effective anesthesia, first available in 1846, followed by the ready availability of antibiotics with the debut of mass-produced penicillin in the 1940s, made more invasive operations safe. Reconstructive and preventive surgeries, now considered routine, were fostered by these landmark events. Slowly, over the decades, the removal of gynecologic organs to treat and prevent female cancers became the accepted standard of care in gynecology that we now take for granted. In this historical context, the Manchester procedure, introduced at the dawn of ether-based anesthesia and years before antibiotics were discovered, was ahead of its time as one of the first soft tissue reconstructive operations designed to treat a non-life-threatening condition.

I was fortunate to learn the Manchester-Fothergill procedure from two of the few masters of this underutilized, uterine-preserving prolapse operation. Its fall into obscurity is most likely related to the evolution of the holy trinity of hysterectomy. Since the 1950s, if a woman is finished making babies and there is any problem with the uterus, cervix or ovaries (fibroids, polyps, heavy bleeding, abnormal Pap smears, ovarian cysts, prolapse), the standard surgical recommendation has typically been to take the uterus out (and usually the ovaries along with it).

At the time the Manchester was fashioned, a British woman born in 1888 could expect to live to the age of 42. In this context the Manchester, as fertility-preserving prolapse repair, made sense. Perhaps local genetic and nutritional factors were causing alarming rates of prolapse in the young women of Manchester, although it is not clear why the surgeons of this region felt compelled to design this operation in an era where surgery was much riskier than it is today.

In modern America, as in most developed nations, severe pelvic prolapse and cervical hypertrophy is much more common in women over 50 than in young women who have yet to give birth. Today, severe prolapse with cervical hypertrophy in young women is relatively rare, being almost always the direct result of childbirth, hence the notion of prolapse repair as a fertility-preservation therapy is practically obsolete. Given the current life expectancy for American women at 80 years, and since common sense dictates that prolapse repair surgery is highly likely to come undone if the woman gives birth after a pelvic reconstructive operation, it became common practice, as life expectancy improved with each generation, to wait until a woman is finished making babies to perform prolapse surgery. In 1888 prolapse repair was done in the hopes that the young woman would still be able to start a family with her uterus "replaced"; by 1998 prolapse repair was routinely delayed until the last baby was born. Waiting until childbearing is completed is assumed to afford each woman the best possible durability of her repair over the remaining decades of her life, something that her turn-of-the-century sister had no such luxury to consider, very likely being dead well before menopause. Given that most modern prolapse repairs are done after completion of childbearing and very often after or near the age of menopause, the contemporary prolapse patient is a prime candidate for the "take it all out" policies still in place in gynecology today. These factors, along with the advent of safe anesthesia and antibiotics, each played a role in promotion of the more invasive hysterectomy over the uterine-preserving Manchester hysteropexy as the solution to uterine prolapse.

As a result of this extirpative philosophy, standard gynecologic training since the 1950s teaches us that uterine prolapse treatment options were limited to two, pessary or hysterectomy, with the Manchester uterine resuspension vanishing, conceptually and practically, as an option in most training centers in this country. Under these influences the Manchester went from an operation used in young women to fix their prolapse while preserving their fertility, to an operation offered in very few centers, reserved, where available, for elderly, sedentary women who needed the quickest, least traumatic operation for prolapse repair. Only recently, with the increasing realization that prolapse repair need not mandate removal of the uterus, has the legacy of the Manchester operation come into full bloom.

#2: Sacrospinous Ligament

These wedge-shaped ligaments, one on each side, attach the sit-bones (ischial tuberosities) to the sacrum bone and are side by side with your sciatic nerves and another important nerve pair called the pudendal nerves.

The pudendal nerves control function and sensation in the anus, the Kegel muscles, the urethra, clitoris and vulva, making the pudendal nerves a very important nerve pair indeed.

The sacrospinous ligaments can be used to anchor and elevate the vaginal cuff (sacrospinous fixation) or the uterus (sacrospinous uterine suspension). Typically only one ligament, usually the right side, is used for sacrospinous prolapse repairs, although some surgeons do suspend to both sides. This operation is done through the vagina.

How long will it last? Sacrospinous fixation of the vaginal cuff (hysterectomy) holds up in 80-90% of patients. Sacrospinous hysteropexy (uterus left in place) success rates are comparable to the hysterectomy-based version, with only 2.3% of patients in one study requiring more prolapse surgery after sacrospinous hysteropexy.

What are the common complications? In another study done by researchers in the Netherlands, women who underwent sacrospinous fixation of the vaginal cuff had higher rates of urinary incontinence than did those who underwent the uterine-sparing sacrospinous uterine resuspension. Sacrospinous fixation also carries a risk of pelvic pain, presumedly from the suture irritating the nearby sciatic nerve, and in some series is associated with rectal complaints as well. Sacrospinous suspensions also pull the top of the vagina to the side to which the suspension is attached, and may reduce the length of the vagina.

#3: Sacrum Bone

The flat bone between the buttocks, the sacrum anchors the bottom of your spine to your tail bone.

Anchored on the front side of this bone (the side you cannot feel through your skin) is the very tip of the most powerful artery in your body, the middle sacral artery of the aorta.

The front side of the sacrum can be used to elevate and anchor the vaginal cuff (sacrocolpopexy) or the uterus (sacrohysteropexy). These suspensions are done abdominally, either through a bikini cut, with the laparoscope, or robotically.

Sacrum suspensions connect either the vaginal cuff or the uterus to the sacrum bone using a strip of graft material. This graft creates a sturdy connection between the vaginal cuff (after hysterectomy) or to the back side of the cervix (for uterine resuspension), bypassing the laxity in the uterosacral ligaments by creating what amounts to a permanent, artificial uterosacral ligament. The graft material varies, from permanent synthetic mesh, a strip of the patient's own connective tissue, or a strip of medically treated connective tissue from an animal donor or human cadaver.

How long will it last? Sacrum suspensions are considered by some reconstructive surgeons to be the most sturdy, with many studies showing success rates of over 90%. When done with the uterus left in, sacrohysteropexy holds up in 93-100% of patients.

What are the common complications? This operation, being abdominal, can take more time in the operating room and can have a longer recuperation than repairs done through the vagina, taking anywhere from 45 minutes to several hours depending on the route of access, be it a bikini-cut incision, laparoscopically or robotically. Adhesions may form between the bowel and the suspension ribbon. On rare occasion hemorrhagic

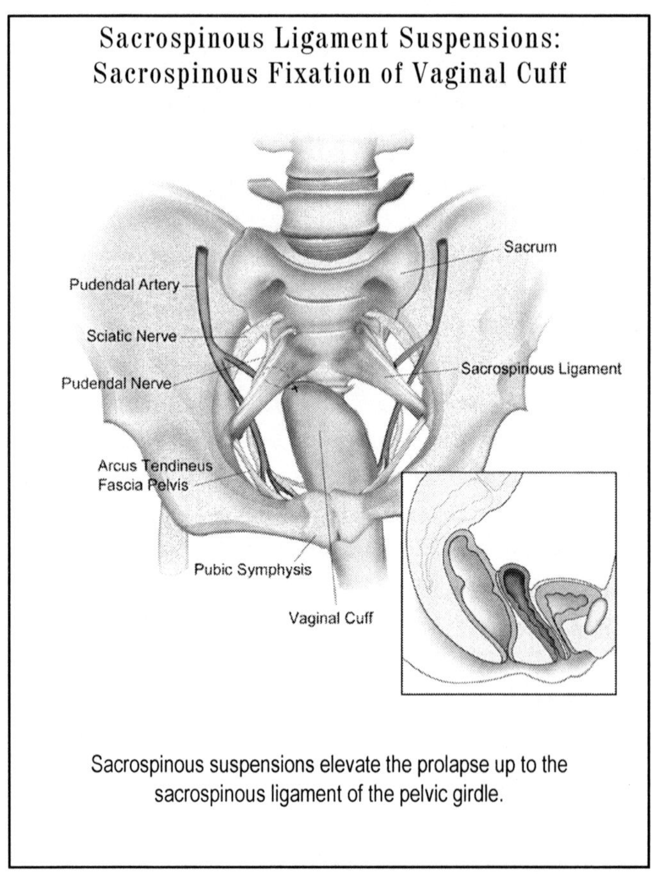

Sacrospinous suspensions elevate the prolapse up to the sacrospinous ligament of the pelvic girdle.

Illustration: Madd Graphix, Inc.

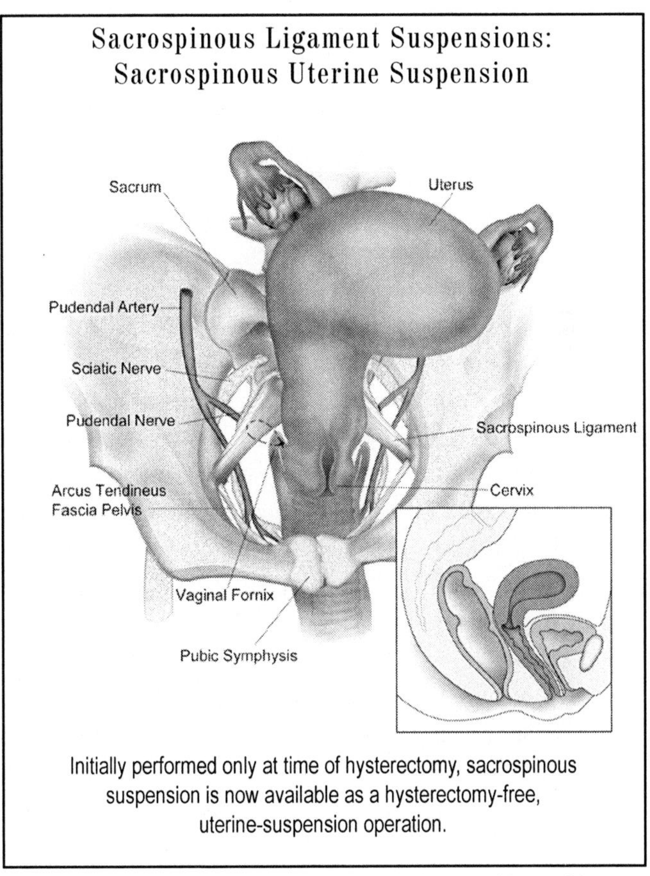

Sacrospinous Ligament Suspensions:
Sacrospinous Uterine Suspension

Initially performed only at time of hysterectomy, sacrospinous suspension is now available as a hysterectomy-free, uterine-suspension operation.

Illustration: Madd Graphix, Inc.

blood loss can occur during this operation, if the middle sacral artery, buried on the front of the sacrum bone in the area of the suspension sutures, is nicked during the procedure. Sometimes the mesh erodes into the top of the vagina or causes delayed-onset problems with the intestines, although one recent study showed no problems with mesh and intestines in a group of women who had this sacrum suspension prolapse repair.

#4: Uterosacral Ligaments

The uterosacral ligaments run inside the pelvis, and are shaped like two open fans, the wide sides arising from the edges of the sacrum bone and the points attaching to the base of the uterus just where it connects to the cervix. These ligaments provide the overwhelming majority of the support to the uterus and top portion of the vagina, with small branches of these ligaments, called the cardinal ligaments, providing the remainder of the support. The uterosacral ligaments function like two robust cables, holding the uterus snugly in place at the top of the vagina.

These uterosacral ligaments can be used to elevate and anchor the vaginal cuff (uterosacral fixation) or the uterus (uterosacral hysteropexy), providing a versatile suspension platform that may be done vaginally, abdominally, laparoscopically or robotically, allowing complete flexibility for each patient's prolapse repair.

Uterosacral suspension shortens the uterosacral ligaments to elevate and support the vaginal cuff or uterus, making it the most anatomically accurate of all these repairs, since the uterosacral ligaments are the body's original support structure of the uterus and uppermost portion of the vagina. The minimally invasive vaginal version of the uterosacral hysteropexy operation restores normal vaginal contour at the same time that it resuspends the uterus in the process (creating a solid anchor for repair of cystocele and rectocele defects below the uterus), holds up well over time, and allows total correction of any prolapse combination without any scars or abdominal incisions.

How long will it last? Uterosacral fixation of the vaginal cuff holds up 90-95% of the time with similar endurance rates when the uterus is left in place, be it laparoscopically or through the other minimally invasive, vaginal approach. The uterosacral suspensions are the most anatomically accurate of the apical suspension techniques, restoring your anatomy to it's original structure.

What are the common complications? It is possible to kink the ureter with uterosacral suspensions, which happens in 1-2% of the cases, making it always advisable for the surgeon to check for this during the operation, so that any kinks can be corrected.

The uterine ligament suspensions are my personal favorite of the uterine prolapse repairs. They may be done by any surgical approach available, be it abdominally or through the vagina. The vaginal uterosacral uterine suspension, shown above, is the operation I designed shortly after my pelvic reconstructive surgery fellowship at New York Presbyterian-Weill Cornell Medical Center in 1995. It offers the advantages of no visible scars and a smooth transition from repairing the prolapsed uterus to repairing any other prolapsed parts at the same operation, such as cystocele, rectocele, vaginal laxity or stress urinary incontinence repair.

Sacrum Bone Suspensions: Sacrocolpopexy of Vaginal Cuff

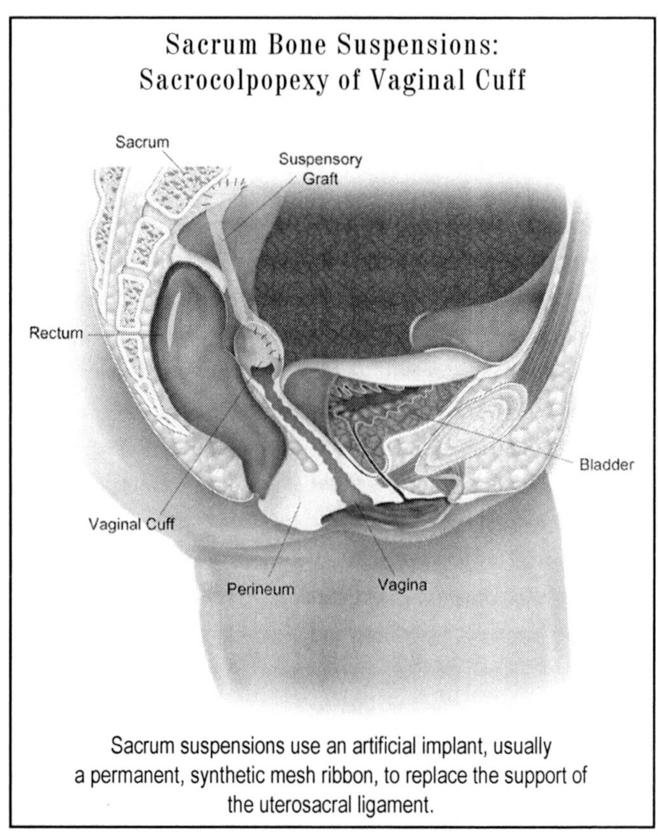

Sacrum suspensions use an artificial implant, usually a permanent, synthetic mesh ribbon, to replace the support of the uterosacral ligament.

Illustration: Madd Graphix, Inc.

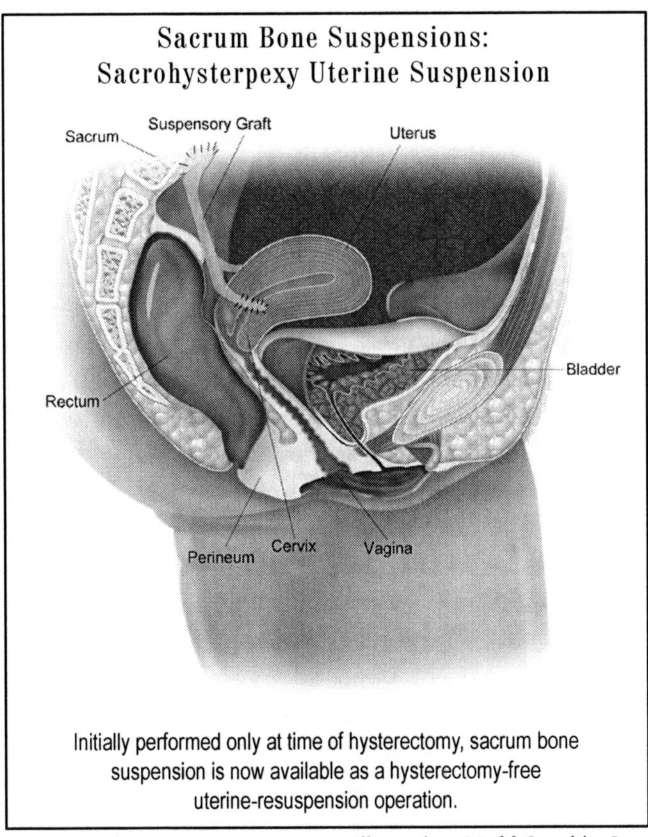

Sacrum Bone Suspensions: Sacrohysterpexy Uterine Suspension

Initially performed only at time of hysterectomy, sacrum bone suspension is now available as a hysterectomy-free uterine-resuspension operation.

Illustration: Madd Graphix, Inc.

The Customer's Always Right

About 14 years ago, I was consultant to a 38 year old divorcee with severe uterine prolapse and vaginal laxity. She was looking for an operation that would preserve the uterus in case she wanted more children and also leave no visible scars that might require explanation to a future husband. Having researched the options, she thought a Manchester procedure would be the best operation for her. Were she 88 instead of 38 I would have agreed, but I was worried that the location of the cervix after a Manchester, typically not lifted quite all the way back up to the top of the vagina, might bother her in a newly minted sexual relationship. With no long term follow-up data on the procedure available in the literature, concerns about Manchester repair durability in a 38 year old were directed to my mentors, who had no experience using it for women in her age range. They both advised me that as far as they were concerned, her best option was a hysterectomy-based vaginal cuff suspension, using a pessary until she was ready to have her uterus removed. Either that, or do a Manchester and take her chances, since neither had ever done one in a young woman who hoped to have more children.

At that time the other three suspensions were only done along with hysterectomy; only the Manchester offered uterine preservation. Sacrohysteropexy (aka sacral uterine suspension), sacrospinous ligament uterine suspension and uterosacral ligament hysteropexy (aka uterosacral uterine suspension) did not exist; only their hysterectomy-based versions (sacrocolpopexy, sacrospinous fixation of the vaginal cuff and uterosacral fixation of the vaginal cuff) were in practice at that time. The first uterus-preserving sacrum bone repair, the sacrohysteropexy, was published in a medical journal in 2001 with the sacrospinous uterine suspension and the uterosacral uterine suspension/uterosacral hysteropexy data following thereafter.

So I fitted her for a pessary. She was back in one month, stating, "I just want to be normal again. I don't want to wear this thing everyday."

And so it went, she would come in, we would review her options, she would leave to come back another time hoping that some new operation had been hatched in the interim. On one of her visits we were going over the operation techniques again when she asked, "can't you do that uterosacral thing through the vagina without removing the uterus?" Bingo. This patient was a genius.

The operation she inspired takes the Manchester "cut-and-wrap" mechanics from a relatively wispy vaginal tuck of the not-so-robust cardinal ligaments, and turns it into a thick belt around the uterus by using a small vaginal incision behind the cervix to access and transpose the insertion of the strong uterosacral ligaments around front for the wrapping portion of the reconstruction. This part of the new operation is exactly like the first step of a vaginal hysterectomy, where the uterosacral ligaments are detached from the back of the cervix. But with this new resuspension, the entirety of the uterosacral ligaments are cut and wrapped around the front of the cervix, as done with the wispier cardinal ligaments during a Manchester but much stronger, functioning like a Heimlich maneuver-type hug, lifting the uterus up and back rather than removing it from the body. Before the Heimlich belt is secured in place, each uterosacral ligament is secured with a stitch halfway between the cervix and the sacrum, just as one does with the original hysterectomy-based uterosacral

Uterosacral Ligament Suspensions: Uterosacral Suspension of Vaginal Cuff

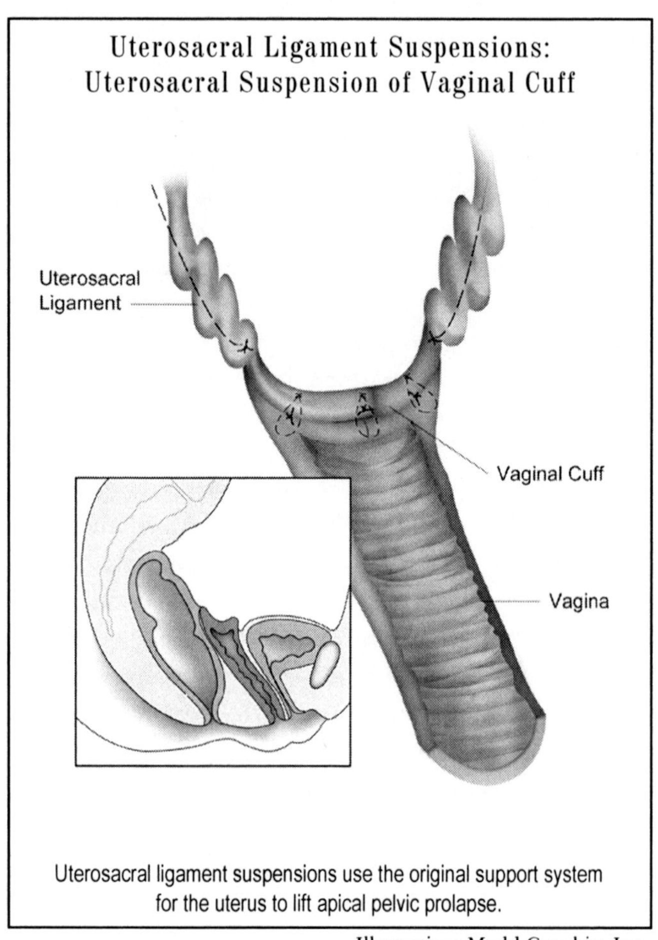

Uterosacral ligament suspensions use the original support system for the uterus to lift apical pelvic prolapse.

Illustration: Madd Graphix, Inc.

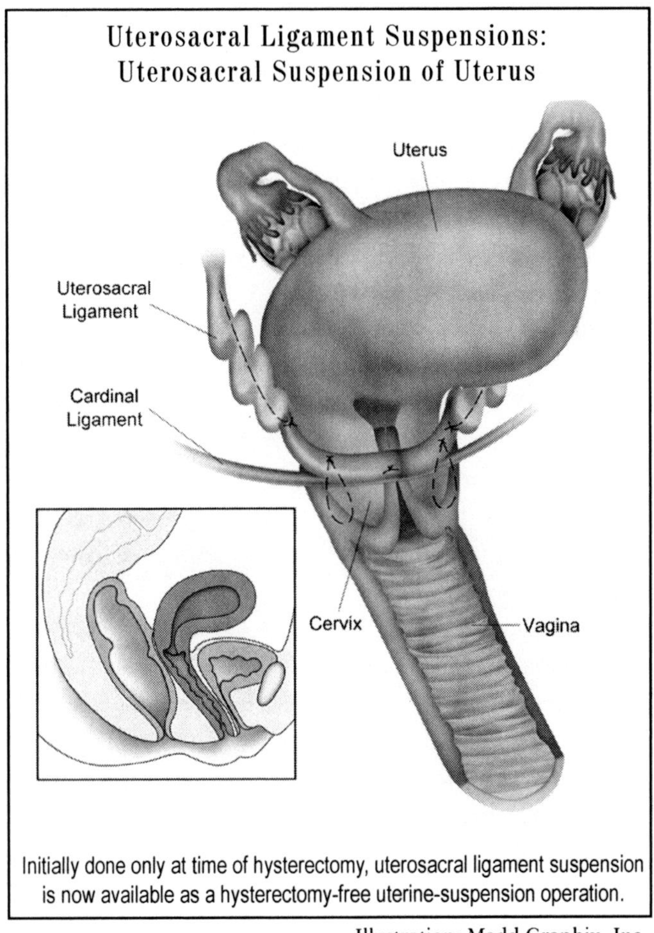

Initially done only at time of hysterectomy, uterosacral ligament suspension is now available as a hysterectomy-free uterine-suspension operation.

Illustration: Madd Graphix, Inc.

suspension of the vaginal cuff. In this new, uterine-preserving modification of the operation, the tucking stitches are placed through the open edge of the back vaginal wall where it was opened behind the cervix, then through the back of the cervix itself, hiking up the cervix/uterus as the stitches, one on each side, are snugly tied.

With any construction it is advantageous to spread out the pressure points over more than one spot, so that gravity and pressure are distributed over a wider surface area. Which works better, walking on snow in high heels or in snowshoes? It's the same idea. Along this structural design concept the vaginal uterosacral hysteropexy combines techniques from two established suspension operations, the double wrap of the Manchester reinforced by a double tuck of the uterosacral suspension. The blending of these two established techniques creates four points of fixation rather than one, spreading the pressure of gravity out over a larger surface area, creating a uterine-suspensory snowshoe.

Unlike the original Manchester operation, the vaginal uterosacral hysteropexy does not include mandatory shortening of the cervix, in which cases the potential for cervical retraction beneath scarred vaginal skin and retained menstrual blood are avoided. The vaginal uterosacral hysteropexy restores the uterus to a normal perch deep in the pelvis where it belongs, without belly scars, unnecessary cervical shortening or the use of synthetic materials.

So Now You Know

...what you need to know to discuss your uterine prolapse repair with your doctor. Traditionally done immediately after removal of the uterus, each of the three suspension techniques, sacrospinous ligament, sacrum bone and uterosacral ligament, are now available in uterine-sparing versions for women who want to avoid hysterectomy.

They all sound great on paper, so how do you decide? These three approaches, sacrospinous ligament, sacrum bone and uterosacral ligament, are all accepted options for the apical portion of any prolapse repair. In the latest gynecologic practice bulletin on pelvic organ prolapse, a thorough review of all available literature for both hysterectomy-based and uterine-sparing operations using any of these three anchor areas showed an overall recurrence rate for apex prolapse (uterus, cervix or vaginal cuff) ranged from 0-20%. The length of follow-up after surgery, the exact combination of procedures, the use of graft material and the age, weight and health of the patients in each series varies, making it impossible to know which one is "the best." Clinical data is important, but at the end of the day, you are an individual, not a case series. First, make sure your surgeon knows about these techniques, and review each one in the context of your particular situation. Then, it's never a bad idea to get a second opinion. Finally, use your common sense and your intuition to tell you if the advice your doctor(s) gave you makes sense for you.

I can tell you that my approach to uterine prolapse is pretty simple: vaginal uterosacral hysteropexy for women who don't need hysterectomy; vaginal hysterectomy with uterosacral fixation of the vaginal cuff for women who do need hysterectomy; abdominal supracervical hysterectomy with abdominal uterosacral suspension of the cervix for women who need a hysterectomy but want the cervix left in place; and abdominal sacrum bone suspension for patients with severe recurrence of uterine or vaginal cuff prolapse. The common denominator for my personal selection process is the utilization of the uterosacral ligament, either your own or a grafted artificial replacement ligament, to resuspend the herniated "ceiling" portion of your prolapse.

All reconstructive surgeons each have their personal philosophies to account for their professional preferences. For instance, no great surprise here, I like the vaginal uterosacral hysteropexy best because it leaves the uterus and ovaries intact, avoids abdominal incisions, is scarless, holds up over time, doesn't require graft material and rarely has a serious complication. And my bias is unavoidable given that I designed the procedure; it's my baby. For women with recurrent prolapse, however, I am inclined to go with the sacrum suspension, which *does* leave belly scars, *does* require graft material, and *is* prone to serious complications, but also bypasses the patient's laxity completely by implanting a durable artificial uterosacral ligament suspension that is, in my opinion, the best option in most cases for patients whose parts fall back down with the less invasive repairs. I personally never do sacrospinous suspensions because they give me the willies, with the vagina pulled over and back onto a ligament it was never originally attached to, right up against the sciatic and pudendal nerves; not my favorite. But, to be fair, I have colleagues who swear that their sacrospinous suspension patients are doing great, loving life, no pain, no problem. For patients, this mix of options and disparity of professional opinions can be the biggest headache of all as they move through the counseling and second opinion maze of surgical decision-making. All these options are

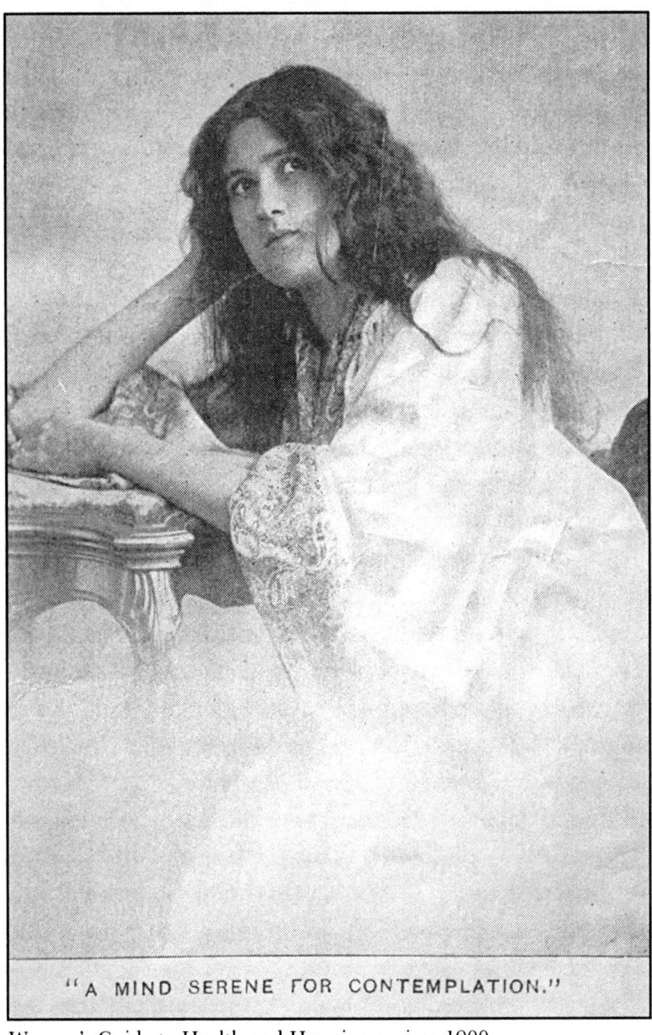

"A MIND SERENE FOR CONTEMPLATION."

Women's Guide to Health and Happiness, circa 1900

accepted standards of care. The key is in formulating the best surgery plan for each individual circumstance.

Ask your surgeon, then ask another surgeon, then ask yourself: does the surgical plan make you comfortable or nervous? If it makes you nervous, keep on looking, and don't take your uterus out unless you have a good reason!

Wait! There's More...

There's more to consider than uterus in/uterus out. If you have pelvic organ prolapse, you most likely have more than one problem. It is most uncommon to find a woman with uterine prolapse who does not also have a cystocele, rectocele, vaginal laxity, urinary incontinence or some combination thereof.

Whatever your personal mixture of prolapsed parts and plumbing problems, fix all of them at the same time, whether you have symptoms from each defect or not. The supports and functions of all these structures are interdependent and one weak link can pull everything out of alignment. For instance, imagine you fix your prolapsed uterus but do nothing about the moderate cystocele (dropped bladder) because your bladder isn't bothering you. Well, symptoms or not, the top of the bladder is connected to the cervix. When the bladder is full it is heavy, like a water balloon, and if it is bulging down into a cystocele, it will pull on your cervix (or top of the vagina if you had hysterectomy) making it more likely that the top of your prolapse repair will come undone. If you fix a cystocele and uterine prolapse but not the rectocele, the rectocele almost always gets worse, eventually bulging so far out that it requires another trip to the operating room to repair. "A stitch in time saves nine" is just as true here as it is for the hem of your dress.

So let's take a look at these other prolapses, starting with dropped bladder repair.

Bladder Lift

Of all the "parts" that might eventually come back down after prolapse repair, bladders are the most likely. Why? Probably because the bladder holds urine, which, like water, is heavy. And the connective tissue that lies in between bladder and vagina, called the "vesicovaginal space," is not particularly robust to begin with. Even in a young woman who has never given birth, this interposing connective tissue layer is about as thick as five sheets of paper. This supportive platform separates vaginal skin from the overlying bladder, sort of like a trampoline. This trampoline connects to the inside of your hip bones to a tendon called the "arcus tendineus fascia pelvis," also called "the white line," just as a real trampoline is connected to its supporting framework. Don't bother to remember the fancy name, just know the "white lines" are there, one on each side, running from front to back, along the inside of your hip bones.

The trampoline can wear out in the center, creating a gap through which the bladder bulges against the elastic vaginal skin. This type of cystocele looks very smooth, just like a balloon, and we call it a "central cystocele." This trampoline can also disconnect from the sides, pulling off of the "white line" inside your hipbones, creating more bulge when you cough, lift, run, etc. We call this a paravaginal cystocele. This type of cystocele usually doesn't feel smooth, the vaginal surface looks crinkled, like cobblestone, and has soft wrinkles belting the bulge horizontally. If you have a cystocele, it may be central, paravaginal, or both central AND paravaginal together.

Paravaginal cystoceles can be repaired through the abdomen (or, as gynecologists say, "from above"), or vaginally ("from below") because it is possible to reconnect the torn vesicovaginal connective tissue back onto the white lines from either approach. With a central cystocele, however, the hole in the middle of the connective tissue between bladder and vagina can only be exposed and closed through the vagina, or "from below." So if you need a cystocele repair, make sure you understand what kind of cystocele you have (central, paravaginal, or both) and how the surgeon plans to fix it.

Fixing cystoceles is a lot like fixing a hernia. Hernia surgeons deal with some of the same issues that reconstructive gynecologic surgeons face; connective tissues are worn away or torn, allowing body parts to bulge into the defect whereever the damaged area may be: the groin, the bellybutton, the diaphragm. Hernias can come back after hernia surgery, not always and not often, but it can happen.

About 10 years ago, graft reinforcement became routine for abdominal hernia operations, and this surgical technique innovation reduced abdominal hernia recurrence rates quite a bit. These implants are thin sheets of body-friendly material that are inserted between the repaired hernia and the overlying abdominal wall to add strength to the repair, making it harder for the hernia bulge to come back. Hernia grafts remind me of "facing" material used by seamstresses and tailors to add support to the collars, lapels and button folds of blouses, jackets, coats and dresses.

Cystoceles, being hernias of the front vaginal wall, allow the bladder to bulge down into the vagina, and are notorious for "coming back down" with the traditional repair techniques of prior decades. These older cystocele repair methods carry recurrence risk up to 30% or greater in some studies. The traditional cystocele repair, called anterior colporrhaphy, relies on a line of tucking stitches in the remnants of connective tissue between bladder and vagina, followed by the trimming of excess vaginal skin underneath the bladder, a structural reinforcement that does nothing whatever about reconnecting bladder support to the "white lines" inside the hip bones.

Over the past eight years, reconstructive pelvic surgical techniques have changed radically, with much attention paid to restoring the "white line" connection in paravaginal cystoceles, and an increasing use of grafts to reinforce the repair of central cystoceles. Prolapse repair graft materials include specially treated skin or body linings from pigs and cows, connective tissue taken from the patient's own body or from cadaveric human donors, absorbable mesh made from a special weave of absorbable surgical suture material, or nonabsorbable permanent synthetic mesh. Whether or not to use graft material, and selecting the right graft for you, is usually based on the severity of the prolapse, your medical history, and your personal philosophy.

For instance, the absorbable grafts are designed to induce your body to lay down solid connective tissue where the graft is inserted so that, eventually, as the graft material dissolves away, the repaired vesicovaginal connective tissue layer is "all you." This sounds great, but must be balanced against a slightly greater probability that the cystocele may recur with absorbable graft than

Central Cystocele

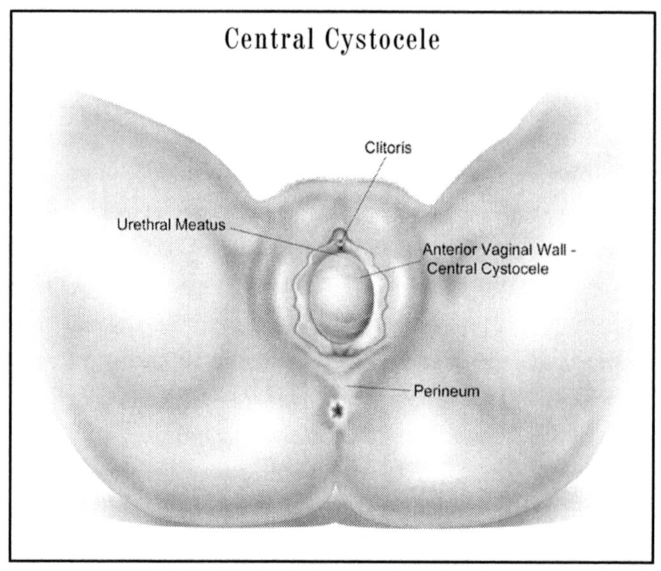

Paravaginal Cystocele

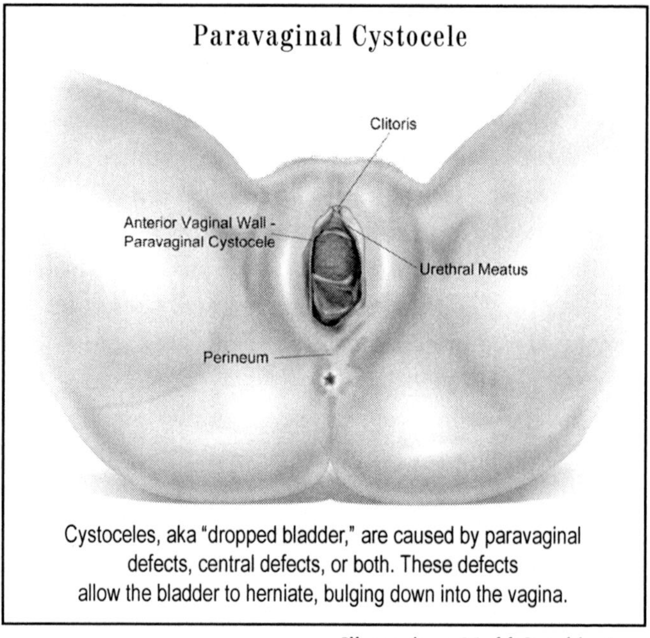

Cystoceles, aka "dropped bladder," are caused by paravaginal defects, central defects, or both. These defects allow the bladder to herniate, bulging down into the vagina.

Illustrations: Madd Graphix, Inc.

with permanent graft. There are no definitive studies comparing permanent and absorbable grafts for pelvic floor reconstruction, making patient counseling an inexact science when it comes to the true and absolute benefit of graft reinforcement and graft selection for pelvic organ prolapse surgery. With graft material interposed between the vagina and bladder, we presume that the possibility of recurrence is lower, similar to the improved durability of abdominal hernias reinforced with graft material. There is growing concern, however, regarding complications associated with the use of graft material in female pelvic reconstruction, particularly with a permanent plastic-type called "polypropylene mesh." These complications lead the FDA to issue a recent warning* detailing growing concerns, including "...erosion of the mesh and scarring of the vagina led to discomfort and pain, including pain during sexual intercourse. Some patients needed additional surgery to remove the mesh that had eroded into the vagina. Other complications included injuries to nearby organs such as the bowel and bladder, or blood vessels."

Personally, I almost always recommend a non-polypropylene graft material when I repair a cystocele, as an insurance policy against the likelihood of cystocele recurrence. The bladder is a water balloon, it's heavy, it's notorious for falling down again, and if you're going to lift it, graft it. Most of the emerging concerns with graft material may be avoided by proper selection and careful technique.

So if you have a cystocele, you want to know if it is paravaginal, central, or both. You want to understand how the approach (abdominal or vaginal) will allow the surgeon to repair the defect(s) causing the cystocele,

*www.fda.gov/cdrh/consumer/surgicalmesh-popsui.html

Rectocele: "Back Wall" Hernia

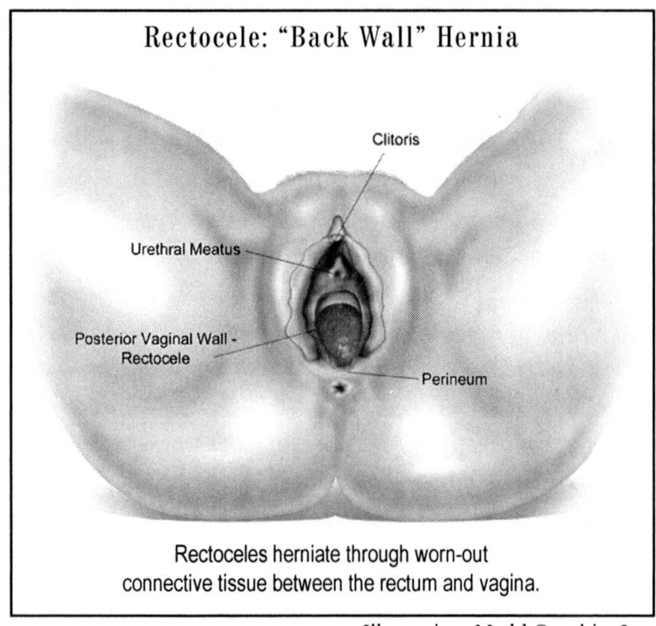

Rectoceles herniate through worn-out connective tissue between the rectum and vagina.

Illustration: Madd Graphix, Inc.

whether or not graft material is wise, what type of graft material your surgeon recommends and why.

Rectal Refurbishment

Rectoceles, unlike cystoceles, are far less likely to recur after repair, and, in my experience, don't always need reinforcing graft material. My personal practice is to use graft material only for rectoceles that have recurred after prior repair, or when the patient has a very large rectum (called a megarectum), a severe, high grade rectocele, or a medical condition that weakens your body's connective tissue, as can happen with severe diabetes, hyperelastic skin conditions, and chronic prednisone therapy, among others, or intractable, chronic constipation. If anything is going to make a rectocele come back after surgery, it is constipation.

There are two basic types of rectocele repair, levatorplasty and site-specific. Levatorplasty is a traditional technique that has recently fallen under scrutiny due to studies showing it may cause chronic pain. In an effort to reduce the risk of chronic pain, the newer "site-specific" repair technique was developed, the benefit of which is a lower rate of chronic pain, but the risk of which is a higher rate of recurrence. Both techniques start out exactly the same; the vaginal skin is carefully dissected (cut away) from the underlying rectum, starting at the vaginal opening and extending to the top of the vagina near the cervix. With the vaginal skin lifted off of the rectum, the rectocele is repaired with levatorplasty or site-specific technique; the excess vaginal skin is trimmed and the edges sewn back together, just like taking in a dart in a skirt or blouse that fits too loosely.

Levatorplasty brings the inside edges of the levator/Kegel muscles closer together in the space between the rectum and vagina, using a series of lacing sutures. Urogynecologists do levatorplasty through an incision in the back wall of the vagina. Our colleagues in colorectal surgery do this exact same procedure through an incision in the front wall of the rectum, reconnecting the levator muscles in the same way but from the other side, which they often use to reinforce rectopexy procedures, (the uterine-resuspension operations of the colorectal world). These two access routes highlight the location of these muscle beds, located between the vagina and rectum in a tissue plane called the rectovaginal space, accessible through either the vagina or the rectum. The levator muscles pull apart with rectocele much as the abdominal muscles pull to the sides of the belly during pregnancy. This muscle separation most often results from stretching during childbirth, or from severe, chronic constipation. Many women with rectoceles have a lot of difficulty doing Kegel exercises; they might contract the muscles very well, but the muscles are so spread apart by the interposing rectocele bulge that it is difficult for the patient to feel any muscle movement. When the edges are brought closer together, the muscles, in my experience, work more efficiently and patients often tell me, "I can Kegel again!"

The key to a good levatorplasty is to avoid making it too tight, or "overcorrecting." If it is too tight, chronic pain may result due to stricture that has to be dilated or loosened surgically. Overcorrection can be avoided in most cases by carefully evaluating the degree of correction of each stitch as you go along during the operation.

The newer, site-specific technique involves opening the back vaginal wall to expose and then close the holes in the rectovaginal connective tissue layer without touching the levator/Kegel muscles. Sometimes the hole is one big one, in which case graft material may be used to cover it, and sometimes the holes are scattered like Swiss cheese, in which case a series of hole-closing stitches restore the connective tissue layer.

To me, the site-specific rectocele repair technique is like the Communist Manifesto: sounds great on paper, but doesn't work very well in real life. Rarely do I "see" the defect in the rectovaginal connective tissue layer; most of the time the connective tissue is completely gone or so patchy and worn away that I wouldn't trust the repair to hold up with site-specific stitching. Additionally, unlike cystocele grafting, graft material in the back wall of the vagina can be a tricky business when it comes to sex after surgery, so I avoid grafting unless I have a good reason to use it in this area.

Reconstructive pelvic surgeons tend toward the passionate when addressing preferences for one technique over another, no less obvious than with the polarized opinions regarding which rectocele repair is superior. Site-specific proponents consider levatorplasty barbaric, and levatorplasty aficionados are known to say things like "site-specific repair is for surgeons who don't know how to do a proper levatorplasty," and so on and so on, at times reminiscent of British legislative sessions, with Lords and Members of Parliament hurling jibes, polite and otherwise, across an antique marble valley. But I digress…

Levatorplasty rectocele repair provides reliable reconstruction without the use of grafts, but may put you at greater risk for adjustments or revisions afterwards to relieve pain and correct any strictures. Site-specific rectocele repair is less likely to cause pain, but tends to recur more often and is more likely to require the use of graft material. So if you have a rectocele, think about which set of pros and cons you prefer, make sure you know which technique your surgeon recommends, and why.

Vaginal Laxity

The perineum is the poor cousin of prolapse repair. This crucial collagen wedge that separates the vaginal opening from the anus is downplayed in surgical textbooks and gynecologic training. When it loses connective tissue, this decreases the thickness of the wedge, causing vaginal laxity, one of several symptoms associated with the condition of perineal atrophy (thinning). Without a cystocele or other flagrantly bulging and prolapsed part(s) above the perineum, it is common for patient complaints to be met with stony forbearance and clinical reassurances that "there is nothing wrong here; you are normal."

The normal structure of the vaginal opening (vulva) includes the labia right next to each other like two parentheses, crowned by the clitoris on top and anchored together at the bottom by a normal, solid perineum. With childbirth, and sometimes just with aging, the perineal connective tissue can thin out and pull sideways into the flesh on either side, taking the bottom of the labia along for the ride, and changing the vulvar shape from two snug parentheses bound together to the abnormal shape of a wide-open triangle, clitoris at the top, with labia pulled to the sides and separated by the widened, thinned-out perineum that forms the base of the triangle. Perineal atrophy (thinning) pulls the labia apart, and brings the anus and vaginal opening closer together.

Thin Perineum: "Vaginal Laxity"

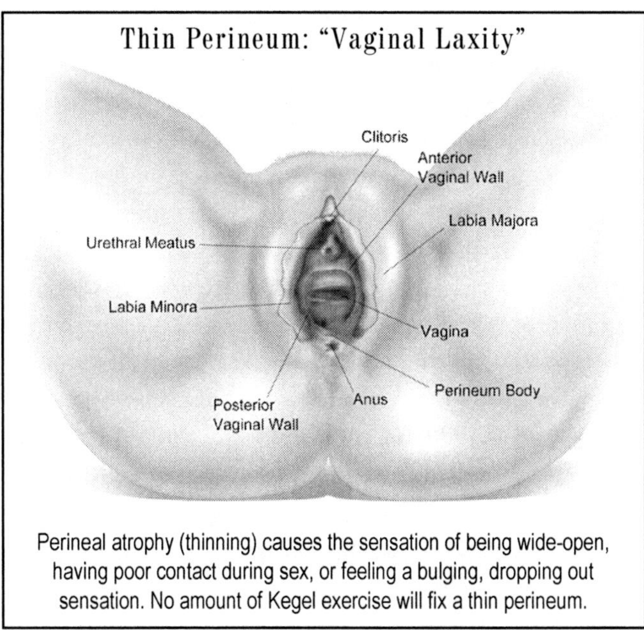

Perineal atrophy (thinning) causes the sensation of being wide-open, having poor contact during sex, or feeling a bulging, dropping out sensation. No amount of Kegel exercise will fix a thin perineum.

After Perineoplasty

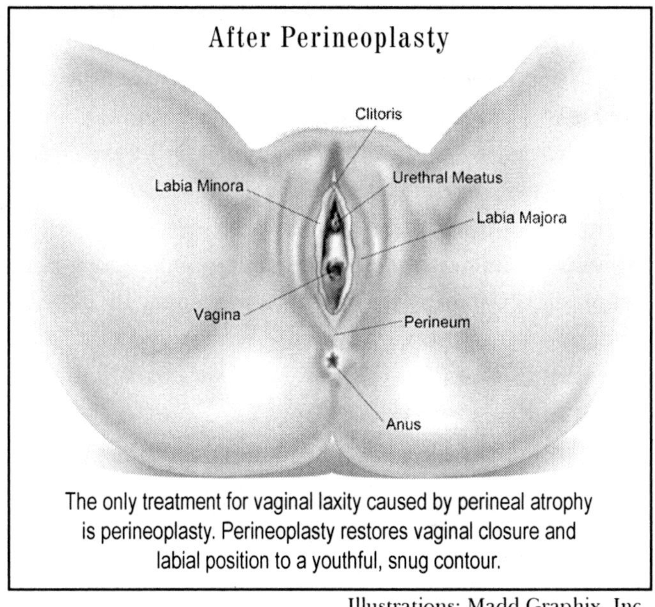

The only treatment for vaginal laxity caused by perineal atrophy is perineoplasty. Perineoplasty restores vaginal closure and labial position to a youthful, snug contour.

Illustrations: Madd Graphix, Inc.

Restoring the perineum, called "perineoplasty," involves a small incision at the bottom of the vaginal opening, through which the perineal connective tissue is carefully put back together in the middle, restoring the normal wedge between vagina and anus.

Of all the types of prolapse defects, perineal thinning is often the most bothersome to the patient, and yet in many a doctor's office, the least acknowledged. Patients complaining of laxity during sex, air trapping in the vagina during yoga class, a terrible "open all the time" feeling, a bizarre falling-out-the-bottom sensation when walking, an inability to close the vagina with Kegel contractions, approach their physicians only to be told "But that's normal. You've had babies, what do you expect?"

While perineal atrophy is common after birthing children, it is not normal, and you need not suffer a life sentence of laxity without reprieve.

If you have perineal atrophy that affects your sexual and physical quality of life, do not be discouraged if your doctor doesn't seem to get it. And don't waste time with exercises; the connective tissue of the perineum won't grow back together if even if you Kegel 500 times a day. Your orgasm may be stronger for all that Kegeling, but the perineum structure can only be corrected with a minimally invasive, ambulatory operation called a perineoplasty. Perineoplasty can be done alone, or in combination with any mix of prolapse repairs you require. If your doctor doesn't understand what you are telling him or her, find one who does.

FOUR

Plumbing

What's worse than a dropped bladder? A dropped bladder that leaks. Not all women with prolapse have leaky bladders, but many who have one problem also have the other. It is tempting to assume that the prolapse is causing the incontinence, and in some cases this may be true; however, not every woman with prolapse leaks urine, and plenty of women wearing incontinence diapers have no prolapse whatsoever. Understanding which came first in a woman with both prolapse and bladder control is not always possible. The good news is, we don't need to know when or why, we just need to know what. What exactly is going on with your prolapse and your bladder? Do you leak too? Or not?

Exert and Squirt

Here's the bottom line: if you have prolapse and a leaky bladder, make sure your doctor figures out exactly why your bladder leaks before you have surgery. If you have the type of leakage called "stress incontinence," this can be fixed at the time of your prolapse repair with a minimally invasive procedure called a sling. Stress incontinence occurs when you "exert and squirt" with a cough or a sneeze, heavy lifting, bending over and the like. It is easily remedied with a urethral sling, a short ribbon of graft material placed between the vaginal skin and the urethra. Slings remind me of bias tape used to reinforce hems and blouse fronts, a crucial detail piece with a big impact on the quality of the garment.

Overactive Bladder

On the other hand, if you have the type of leakage called "urge incontinence" or "overactive bladder," you may need special bladder retraining and pelvic floor physical therapy or medications after prolapse surgery. A sling, which is only for "exert and squirt" stress incontinence, does nothing for women with overactive bladder.

However, one third of incontinent women have both stress and urge incontinence, in which case you'll be helped in part by the sling, but may still need overactive bladder treatment after you recuperate from the surgery.

If you have prolapse and don't leak, I have news for you. Some women with prolapse have stress incontinence but don't know it. Normally, urine is prevented from constantly flowing out of the bladder by the sphincter around the urethra. The sphincter squeezes the urethra shut tight at all times except when urinating; when you urinate the urethral sphincter relaxes so the urine can pass through into the toilet. Stress incontinence is caused by a weak urethral sphincter. Think of it as a gasket that may not last a lifetime.

The female urethra is a short tube about 2-3 inches in length. It's male equivalent is contained within the body of the penis and is, hopefully, several times longer than the female version. In men the urethra is a long straw and in women it's a short straw. With severe prolapse, the urethra can be kinked or compressed just like bending or stepping on a garden hose or kinking or squeezing a soda straw. Anything that kinks or compresses the urethra can mask urethral weakness, literally hiding the incontinence condition. In fact, many women with severe prolapse actually complain of bladder problems at the opposite side of the spectrum, struggling with incomplete bladder emptying and a slow, dribbling stream that keeps them on the toilet seat far too long.

With prolapse repair, any urethral compression and kinking is also corrected, restoring urine flow and bladder emptying to normal. This unkinking also will unmask any preexisting, hidden urethral sphincter weakness, leaving the poor patient cured of her prolapse only to be cast into the equally mortifying world of urinary incontinence.

It is simple to find out whether or not you have this prolapse-concealed (occult) stress urinary incontinence. With your bladder very full, your doctor can hold the prolapsed parts in proper position, where they will be after surgery, and check you for leaking while you cough and strain. If you don't leak lying down, double-check with the same procedure while standing up. If you don't leak with a full bladder with the prolapse held in proper position, either on the exam table or standing up, you most likely do not have hidden (occult) stress incontinence and prolapse repair is all that is needed. If you DO leak with this test, you probably WILL leak after prolapse surgery unless a urethral sling, or some other stress incontinence

Stress Incontinence: "Exert and Squirt"

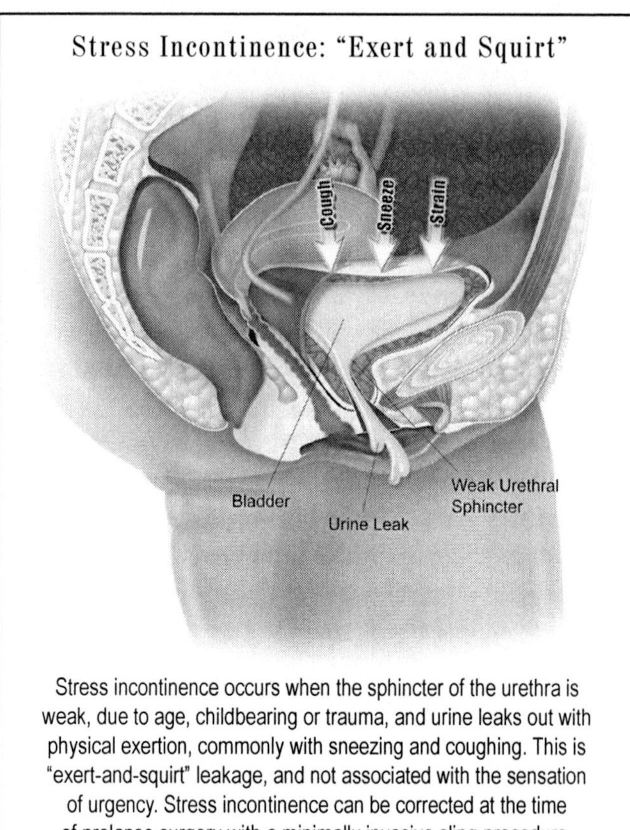

Stress incontinence occurs when the sphincter of the urethra is weak, due to age, childbearing or trauma, and urine leaks out with physical exertion, commonly with sneezing and coughing. This is "exert-and-squirt" leakage, and not associated with the sensation of urgency. Stress incontinence can be corrected at the time of prolapse surgery with a minimally invasive sling procedure.

Illustration: Madd Graphix, Inc.

Urge Incontinence: "Overactive Bladder"

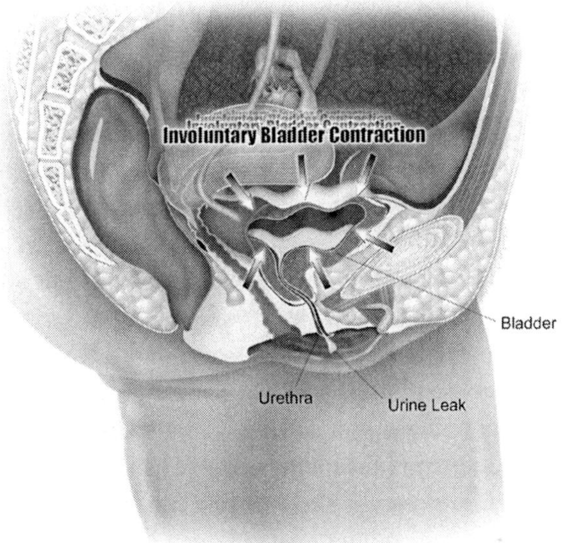

Urge incontinence occurs when the bladder contracts involuntarily, as in a bladder spasm, and the bladder evacuates, much as it does on the toilet. The primary symptom of urge incontinence is urgency, a sudden compelling need to urinate that is difficult or impossible to control. Commonly referred to as "wetting my pants," urge incontinence may not always calm down after cystocele repair.

Illustration: Madd Graphix, Inc.

procedure, can be done at the same time as your prolapse repair. Slings, which used to take an hour to do, now take 15 minutes using new, minimally invasive devices that look just like curved upholstery needles. If you need a urethral sling for exert-and-squirt leaking, it's easy to add on to your operation, and it won't make the surgery or recuperation harder or longer.

In other words, make sure that your doctor figures out: do you only need renovations (prolapse repair), or do you need plumbing (urethral sling) *and* renovations?

If you wet yourself because of an overactive bladder, or "urge incontinence," a sling will not help you, in fact it could make your overactive bladder worse. If the overactive bladder does not calm down with cystocele repair, you may need to use medications or sign up for combined Kegel exercise therapy and bladder retraining drills.

After walking and talking, toilet training is one of the biggest accomplishments many of us will ever achieve, and when any one of these bodily functions is lost, the impact goes beyond the physical deep into the psyche. In other words, wetting your pants not only is messy and not normal, it can drive you nuts and ruin your self-esteem, your social life, your athletic performance, your professional presence and your sexuality. If you have prolapse and you're contemplating surgery, make sure that your surgeon takes your bladder as seriously as you do. Assume nothing. Or as my childhood upholstery magician used to say through pursed, pin-filled lips, "Measure twice, cut once."

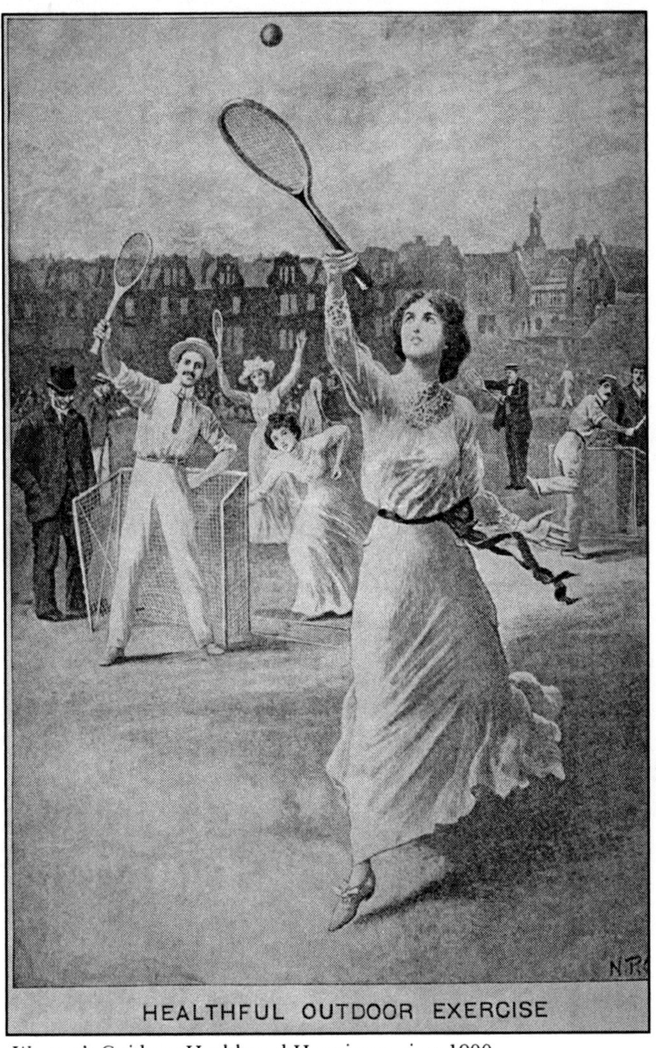

Women's Guide to Health and Happiness, circa 1900

FIVE

Rejuvalicious

Pregame Prep

The success of reconstructive pelvic surgery involves an integrated selection of procedures to repair all defects, and the integrity of the wound healing after the surgery is completed; both factors are critical. Integral to a successful outcome is attitude. That's right, attitude. In my experience, patients who are upbeat and positive about their reconstructive surgery have speedier, more comfortable recuperations than do patients who feel victimized by their condition and fearful or angry about the planned operation. I often tell patients to treat the operation as an athletic event. The day of the operation is "game day," and their role in preparing for surgery and recuperation affects the outcome. So what can you do to improve your outcome other than show up in the operating room on the appointed day?

First, if you smoke, STOP. Healing uses a lot of oxygen from your blood stream and is ultimately delivered to the healing areas in the tiny vessels called capillaries. Capillary blood flow is severely damaged in smokers, reducing oxygen delivery to the body's tissues, and as a result, they are notorious for not healing well. Similarly, if you are diabetic, asthmatic, hypertensive, or have any other chronic medical condition, make sure you are under good control before and after the operation. High blood sugar, for instance, inhibits the transport of fibroblasts, the cells that produce the collagen of wound healing, reducing connective tissue density and the overall quality and integrity of the healing tissues.

Exercise stimulates blood flow, growth hormone production and endorphins, all of which stimulate the healing process, so come into your operation in the best shape you can manage. Kegel regularly so that the muscles around the repair are in the best shape possible. If you cannot Kegel because the muscles are too weak, you may need to use biofeedback or even wait until after the surgery to start a Kegel fitness program. But if you *are* able to Kegel before the surgery, make that a part of your preparations.

Nutritional supplements improve wound healing. My patients take some or all of the following: a good multivitamin along with 500 mg L-carnitine, 1 gram of arginine, 30 mg zinc, and 500 mg extra vitamin C, each of which is an established wound-healing booster well documented in the medical literature. Also, topical estrogen has been shown to help wound healing both in men and women, and certainly helps healing in the vagina, so women who are estrogen depleted from menopause start fingertip application of estrogen cream applied to the vaginal opening before surgery, continuing on again after surgery.

If you suffer with constipation, you must get your &@!% under control before the operation, even if you have to use stimulant laxatives temporarily. Start with 2 tablespoons of flaxseed per day (you can put this in your cereal, yogurt, peanut butter, soup, whatever) and 400 mg Magnesium oxide. A pre-surgery consultation with a gastroenterology dysmotility specialist may be a good idea if your constipation is long-standing or severe. Straining at stool is not good for the repair.

I instruct most patients do a bowel prep before surgery, a total colon cleanout just like the prep for colonoscopy. Your surgeon may not require this, but I find it improves visualization for the uterine resuspension, improves the safety and integrity of the rectocele repair, and reduces postoperation gas pain and constipation; you can't be constipated right after surgery if there's nothing inside your intestines to be constipated with.

Be realistic in your expectations. Even though it is minimally invasive and, when done vaginally, leaves no visible scars, complex prolapse repair is a big operation. The uterus, cervix, bladder, urethra, anus, rectum, perineum and Kegel muscles are all affected. Your body's healing process will take a lot of energy. You will be tired, you may have a few days of mild depression in the first week or two, and for a couple of weeks you will be in a position where the only person you can take care of is yourself. This is a difficult thing for many women to accept. Accept it already, put yourself first. I promise you that the world will not stop rotating on its axis if you are not on your A–game for a few weeks. Stock up on comedy flicks, good books and healthy, easy fix meals. We're talking pain killers, naps, baths and snacks. You can do it.

Game Day

Prolapse repair involving combined defects typically takes 1-3 hours in the operating room. Anesthesia options include either epidural/spinal anesthesia with sedation, or general anesthesia where you are connected to a respirator. I prefer the epidural unless there is a good reason to avoid your spine.

After the operation, most patients spend one or two nights in hospital followed by two weeks of minimal activity at home; you can walk and take care of yourself, but housework, chores and commuting are out. I encourage patients to take a month off if they can. Some women need an extra week or two before the fatigue of healing fades away. At minimum, plan for a two-week break from your normal activities.

Prolapse repair of single defects, such as perineoplasty or urethral sling for leakage, are completely different in terms of recuperation. They take a half hour on the operating room table, you usually go home the same day, and you can return to full activities (except sex) within a week in most cases. Single-defect repairs can be done under short-acting spinal or local anesthesia with sedation, also called "twilight" anesthesia.

Recovery

At home, continue your wound-healing supplement regimen. Bathing with Epsom salts will relax the muscles in the lower back and pelvis, improve blood flow and help the sutures to dissolve. You can bathe within 48 hours of the surgery. You will find yourself easily fatigued, your body's signal that it is busy healing, so give it some help with frequent naps. After a few days start light exercise, short walks, gentle stretching, isometrics and massage, all helpful during the first two weeks.

If you are asthmatic, suffer terrible allergies or catch a cold while you're recuperating, suppress the coughing and sneezing with medication. Repetitive coughing and sneezing will strain the sutures. Ditto with constipation; constipation is against the rules. Do whatever you have to do to avoid straining at stool during the healing period.

Despite my warnings about fatigue and downtime, many women actually feel pretty good a lot sooner than I describe in preoperation counseling, and that's great, but you still have to take it easy for the first few weeks in order to set yourself up for the best possible wound healing. Wound healing is a complicated process that actually takes a full year.

The first phase of wound healing involves blood clotting at all incision sites and the migration of inflammatory cells that release proteins and other particles to attract the all-important fibroblast cells (they make collagen) to the healing area. This takes place over the first day or so, and during this time you will have the worst of the pain. This is why most patients with complex repairs stay in hospital for a day or two; you'll want to, trust me.

The second phase takes place over the first month after the operation. Called the proliferative phase of wound healing, it is the time when the fibroblast cells lay down all your new collagen. This collagen is fresh and new; it needs to "set," think "firm Jell-O™" or "elastic cement." This brand new collagen is the key to your new pelvic support system. If during this time you are jumping on the trampoline or sneezing your head off with allergies, you may disrupt the integrity of the collagen architecture. If you are smoking two packs per day or not getting enough rest, you may not make good collagen in the first place.

Over the ensuing year this new collagen remodels by cross-linking, gaining strength (hopefully) and smoothing out, kind of like ironing a wrinkled sheet. This final "remodeling" phase is very obvious with surface scars, where the incision line visibly fades from pink or dark brown to baseline skin tone, flattening and softening in the process. So be healthy and take it easy for a few weeks. It's the smart thing to do.

Making It Last

"Funny, that's what he said last night..." But seriously, once you've gone through a prolapse repair, there are some wise habits you'll want to adopt.

First, make Kegel exercise part of your daily routine. These muscles are the backup scaffolding for the vagina. You may find that Kegels are easier to do and feel stronger once your organs are back where they belong. For patients with skinny or weak levator muscles I recommend postoperation exercise programs using biofeedback and painless electric stimulation. These workout programs come under the heading "pelvic floor physical therapy." It's just like working out with a personal trainer. Your surgeon may offer this therapy in his or her office, or you may use a physical therapy center that has a pelvic floor specialist on staff. Most patients need 4-8 weeks of sessions to get into good shape. You work out during the weekly session, then work at home with personally tailored exercise regimens on days in between sessions. Consider being fitted for a Colpexin device, which both supports vaginal structure and passively exercises the levator muscles as you go about your day. Kegel exercise, the dental floss of feminine fitness, is the lifelong habit of choice between your navel and your knees.

Annual pelvic support checkups are the best way to keep an eye on the durability of the repair. Exam table and standing evaluation of uterine, bladder and rectal support and perineal body structure are most easily done at the time of your annual gynecology visit, or as a separate visit to the reconstructive surgeon. Either way, have a doctor keep an eye on your insides. The earlier you find a recurrence, the easier the revision and recuperation. And if prolapse never recurs, you'll feel better knowing that everything is exactly as it was right after the surgery.

Avoid heavy lifting, and when you do lift, use good lifting body mechanics. There are no specific guidelines for lifting after prolapse repair. I recommend a generic 30 lbs lifting limit, exclusive of picking up children and unavoidable lifts. This lifting limit rule also benefits your knees, ankles and back.

Avoid constipation. Impacted stool can stretch out the back wall of the vagina, causing a rectocele to recur. Straining at stool can weaken all of the supports, putting you at risk for uterine or vaginal prolapse, cystocele and rectocele.

Stay fit. Sports and workouts stimulate growth hormone, which keeps your connective tissue metabolism well-balanced and youthful. Choose non-jarring activities if you can: race walk or bike instead of running, elliptical machine instead of treadmill, bungee jumping rather than parachute jumping. I'm not making this up; data from the United States Army show that young women paratroop trainees, none of whom had any children yet, were much more likely to develop moderate prolapse by the end of their paratrooper (parachute) training as compared to the regular trainees. According to these investigators, it was clear that "The forces transmitted to the female pelvis during paratrooper training are significant and cause pelvic support defects."[1] Tai Chi, anyone? Incorporate Kegel counter-contractions into your gym workouts, particularly during weight lifting and abdominal exercises. Remember to exhale when exerting yourself.

Kegels, pelvic support checkups, safe lifting technique, good bowel habits, and fitness; why wait until you need surgery? Start now!

1 Larsen WI, Yavorek T. Pelvic prolapse and urinary incontinence in nulliparous college women in relation to paratrooper training. Int Urogynecol J Pelvic Floor Dysfunct 2007.

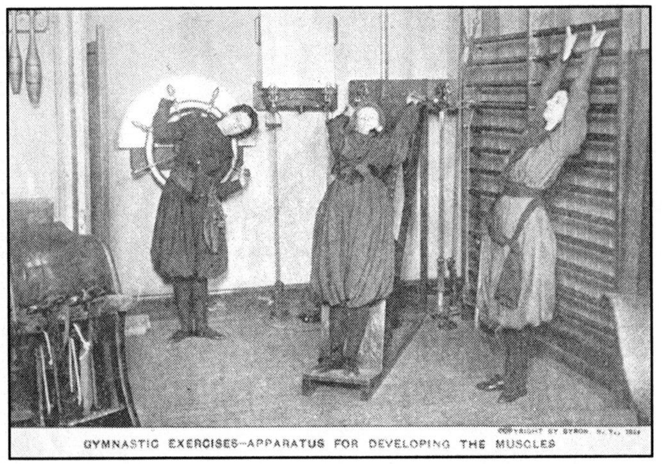

GYMNASTIC EXERCISES—APPARATUS FOR DEVELOPING THE MUSCLES

Women's Guide to Health and Happiness, circa 1900

Epilogue

New Tricks

Urogynecology is a new clone of an old dog, a puppy with a lot of great new tricks, and just in time, I'd say. All that prolapse is damned depressing, but less depressing than it was decades ago when the only repair work available was done by surgeons who were more concerned with taking your parts out than putting them back in place, with no clue about white line repairs, or graft materials, hidden incontinence or body-image issues after motherhood. And who treated prolapse repair as a last-resort option to be doled out frugally and only to women who were, literally, falling apart.

The Plumbing and Renovations of Vaginal Rejuvenation

I interact regularly with beloved colleagues who speak of vaginal laxity repair as if it was the height of cosmetic surgical lunacy, considered normal only in those bicoastal capitals of vanity, Los Angeles and New York, where, allegedly, "nothing is really real." The rest of the country's women, these out-of-town colleagues inform me, have a more reasonable take on laxity and prolapse, or as one colleague held forth, "It's like an old sweater, not as tight as it used to be, a hole in the elbow and a stain or two, a little faded, but it's comfortable. Why mess with it?" And that's fine. Comfy old sweaters should not be messed with, I agree. But pullovers where the hole for the head is as wide as the waistband deserve a little tailoring, whether you're strolling on Melrose, cooking Cajun in bayou country, chillaxing in Tribeca, or sweating it out in the middle of a Nebraskan soy bean field. Unless, of course, the head going through that hole (ahem) *needs* all that room... I'm just saying. It's nice to have options, and it's nice to know what those options are, and it's nice to be able to get your parts fixed if you want to. Or not. Your call.

It's nice to have a user-friendly label for all these maneuvers, a label that resonates with real women living real lives, unveiling some long guarded secrets of the gynecologic gate-keepers. That label is vaginal rejuvenation, and it is to "Oh my Lord I could park a truck down there! Everything's out of place. Where can I go for help?" what Urogynecology is to Gynecology. Vaginal rejuvenation, a user-friendly signpost to women in need of plumbing and renovations, is neither demon nor darling. It's a choice.

The Price Tag on Choice

The flip side of any choice is responsibility. Doctors have the responsibility of sorting out the medically necessary from the purely cosmetic and the medically unproven, giving you the opportunity to grasp the differences between the three and the risks, benefits and alternatives to any procedure you may consider. You have a responsibility to carefully consider all your issues while you contemplate all your options. Take a look at your motivations. Are you desperate to save your relationship and hoping that an operation will do the trick? Or are you in a stable, loving situation with one nagging physical problem that is throwing an otherwise wonderful intimacy off track? Are you looking to revise a body part for your own comfort and confidence? Or are you responding to the cruel comments of an unworthy partner? Whether you call it vaginal rejuvenation or reconstructive pelvic surgery, operations to restore feminine anatomy are no substitute for healthy self-esteem or couples counseling. If your personal life is strained due to infidelity or abuse, no operation under any label will make that relationship better. Many's the time I sat in Obstetrics clinic with a 20-something year old woman after birthing her first six pound baby, handing her tissues as she wept that her husband was cheating on her because "My vagina's too loose. So he goes out with other women. Make me tighter." You get my point. In surgical training the standard line is "the chance to cut is the chance to cure," which is a hell of a lot of fun to say when you want to bait your nonsurgical colleagues, but in real life, a scalpel cuts both ways, good and bad. Before you go under the gynecologic knife, make sure it's for the right reasons.

Putting Prolapse in Perspective

Prolapse is an uncomfortable word, inducing visions of body parts flopping about and not staying put, and in severe prolapse, that is, unfortunately, a fairly accurate image. Mild and moderate prolapse, however, is far from "floppy," rather being a variant of normal, more accurately described as internal vaginal laxity. In one recent study, mild to moderate prolapse was found to be minimally or not at all symptomatic. If it's not bothering you, it's not a problem. So the researchers kept an eye on these women over the next few years to see what happened, and in almost 3%, the prolapse actually regressed in a significant way. 10% of the study participants, unfortunately, progressed a lot, and the remaining participants stayed about the same or regressed/progressed just a little, leading the researcher to the surprising conclusion that "mild pelvic organ prolapse is a fluid state."[1] Women who came in with greater degrees of prolapse, were overweight or had birthed more children were more likely to progress.

Good news! A little bit of pelvic laxity now does not mean you will definitely have severe prolapse in the future; in fact, quite the opposite may transpire. So no panicking if your doctor tells you that you have a small cystocele and a little bit of a rectocele—that's practically normal. Do your Kegels and move on.

On the other hand, if you do have severe prolapse, it is not a badge of failure. Female pelvic prolapse is a by-product of childbearing, elastic connective tissue and vigorous living. It is a sign that you have lived a full and, literally, upright life. It is not your fault, it is not some-

1 Bradley CS, Zimmerman MB, Qi Y, Nygaard IE. Natural history of pelvic organ prolapse in postmenopausal women. Obstet Gynecol 2007; 109(4):848-54

thing you have to live with, and it is not a problem that hysterectomy will fix.

In 1940 an American woman could expect to live a few years past menopause to the age of 59. If you lived long enough to develop vaginal prolapse, just about any operation was likely to last a lifetime, in large part because life expectancy was so short. Add to this environment the rudimentary treatments for gynecologic cancer of that time, and you can understand how the 'hysterectomy-as-cancer-prevention" rule made a lot of sense back in the day.

Today the most rapidly growing segment of the population are people over 80, the majority of whom are women with unprecedented lifestyles and quality-of-life expectations compared to prior generations. One of these expectations is choice. Women are no longer willing to undergo hysterectomy unless it is the best choice. When it comes to prolapse repair, other issues aside, hysterectomy is not mandatory, no matter how severe the prolapse and no matter how far past childbearing you may be. The choice is yours. Choose wisely.

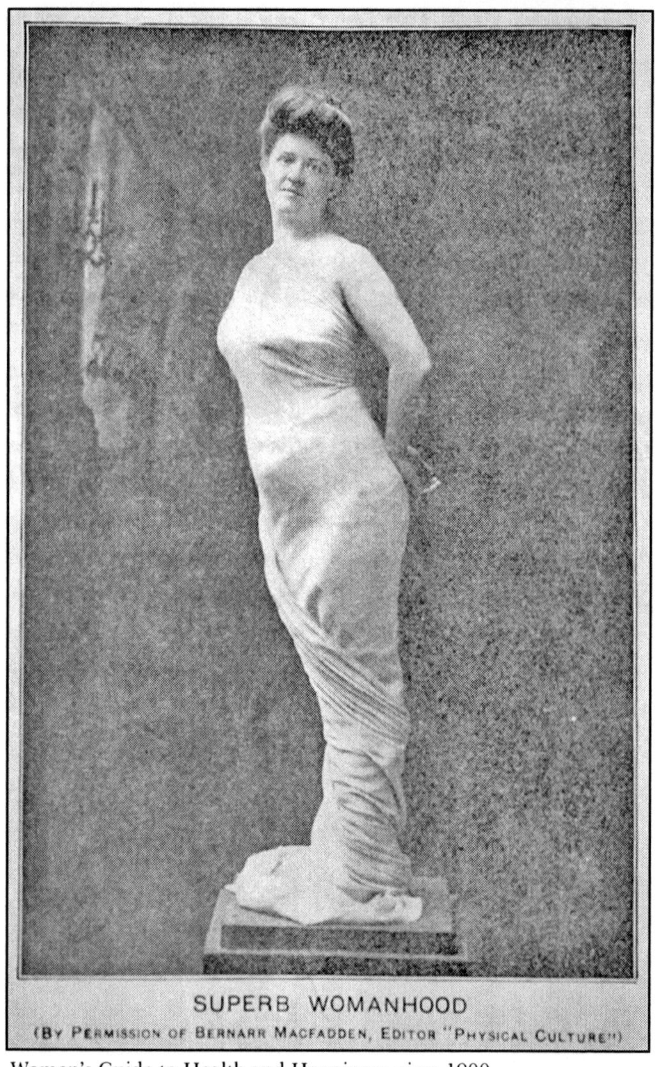

SUPERB WOMANHOOD

(By Permission of Bernarr Macfadden, Editor "Physical Culture")

Women's Guide to Health and Happiness, circa 1900

Glossary

Adenomyosis: Uterine condition where the lining of the uterus becomes thick and spongy and erodes into the muscular wall of the uterus. It may cause uterine enlargement and heavy vaginal bleeding.

Adjunctive: With regards to medical treatments, adjunctive treatments are complementary, or in addition, to the main therapy.

Arcus Tendineus Fascia Pelvis: Dense connective tissue band running inside each of the hip bones that contributes to support of the bladder, levator muscles and other pelvic organs.

Anus: The opening of the rectum that controls bowel movements.

Biofeedback: A therapeutic technique used to improve pelvic muscle coordination and strength that involves visualizing pelvic muscle activity on a computer monitor.

Bladder: The organ that stores urine located behind the pubic bone and in front of the uterus.

BRCA gene: A gene related to tumor growth, often inherited, that makes the woman much more vulnerable to breast and ovarian cancer.

Cadaver: A dead body preserved for dissection related to medical teaching or research. Cadaveric: from a dead body.

Central cystocele: A dropped bladder caused by a thinning or absence of connective tissue support between the bladder and the front vaginal wall.

Cervical hypertrophy: Thickening and elongation of the cervix most commonly associated with uterine prolapse.

Cervix: The opening of the uterus into the vagina.

Coccyx: Tailbone, located below the sacrum and directly in back of the rectum.

Collagen: Fibrous connective tissue made of protein, produced by fibroblast cells, found in all bodily connective tissue.

Colorectal surgery: Reconstructive surgical specialty that focuses on diseases and conditions of the gastrointestinal tract.

Colpexin: A vaginal device that supports mild to moderate prolapse and exercises the levator muscles.

Colporrhaphy: Prolapse operation that lifts a dropped bladder (anterior colporrhaphy) or fixes a bulging rectum (posterior colporrhaphy) by using a line of tucking stitches.

Cystocele: Dropped bladder due to tearing or thinning of the connective tissue that supports the bladder and front vaginal wall.

DES: Diethyl Stilbestrol, an estrogen-type medication used decades ago to prevent miscarriages, withdrawn from the market when found to increase cancer risk in the daughters of women who took it during pregnancy.

Dysmotility: Hyperactive or slow intestinal motility that can be associated with diarrhea or constipation.

Extirpation (extirpative): With regard to surgery, procedures that involve removal of organs or tissues, as opposed to reconstructive operations.

Fascia: Formed connective tissues of the body, present in sheetlike layers and in ligaments and tendons.

Female urology: The subspecialty within urology that focuses on urinary tract and prolapse problems.

Fembrace: Girdle-style device designed to support severe pelvic organ prolapse.

Fibroblasts: The cells in the body that produce collagen, the body's connective tissue fibers.

Fibroids: Noncancerous smooth muscle tumors, often found in the uterus, tubes and ovaries.

Gastroenterology: The medical specialty that treats problems of the esophagus, stomach and intestines.

Hysterectomy: Surgical removal of the uterus and cervix.

Hysteropexy: Uterine resuspension that lifts a prolapsed uterus back into normal position.

Ischial tuberosities: The prominent portion of the pelvic bones that bear most of your weight when seated.

Kegel exercise: As per Dr. Arnold Kegel, these strengthen the levator muscles in the pelvis.

Kidney: The organs that filter the blood and produce urine, connected to the bladder by the ureter.

Levator muscles: Pelvic muscles that wrap around the bladder, vagina and rectum.

Levatorplasty: A method of repairing rectoceles that utilizes the levator muscles that can be done through the posterior vaginal wall or the anterior rectal wall.

Middle sacral artery: A small blood vessel that arises from the bottom of the aorta, running along the anterior surface of the sacrum and coccyx bones of the spine.

Onanism: A synonym for masturbation (and coitus interruptus), derived from the story of Onan in the Book of Genesis, who was slain for committing the sin of "wasting his seed upon the ground."

Oophorectomy: Surgical removal of the ovaries.

Ovary: Reproductive organ that releases eggs for fertilization and secretes sex hormones into the bloodstream.

Paravaginal cystocele: A dropped bladder caused by a lateral tearing or disruption of the connective tissue support layer between the bladder and the front vaginal wall where it connects to the inside of the hip bones.

Pelvic organ prolapse: Umbrella term that refers to all types of prolapse such as dropped bladder, bulging rectum, vaginal laxity and uterine prolapse.

Perineal atrophy: Thinning of the connective tissue between vagina and anus often associated with the sensation of vaginal laxity.

Perineoplasty: Operation to repair vaginal laxity.

Perineum: The connective tissue wedge between vagina and anus.

Pessary: Vaginal support device to hold up pelvic organ prolapse.

Pudendal nerve: The pelvic nerve, one on each side, that supplies the vulvar structures, urethral and anal sphincters and levator muscles.

Rectocele: Rectal bulge caused by weakening of connective tissue in the pelvis.

Rectopexy: A colorectal operation to lift a prolapsing or redundant rectosigmoid colon.

Rectovaginal space: The area between the front wall of the rectum and back wall of the vagina.

Rectum: The section of the intestines between the vagina and the tailbone just above the anus.

Sacrospinous ligament: The dense, wedge-shaped pelvic ligament that connects the sacrum bone to the ischium bone.

Sacrum: The large triangular shaped bone at the bottom of the spine, above the tailbone (coccyx) and in between the hip bones.

Sciatic nerve: A very large nerve that runs from the area underneath the buttock muscles down the back of the leg, supplying the thigh, leg and foot.

Ureter: Tube that transports urine from the kidney to the bladder.

Urethra: Controls urination, opening of the bladder.

Urethral sling: Operation to treat stress (exert and squirt) urinary incontinence.

Urethral sphincter: The bladder's control mechanism, partly involuntary and partly voluntary.

Urogynecology: The subspecialty within gynecology that focuses on bladder and rectal function, pelvic organ support and childbirth-related conditions.

Uterine prolapse: Descent of the uterus caused by laxity in the connective tissue supports in the pelvis.

Uterosacral ligaments: Connective tissue bands that hold the uterus in place.

Uterus: Reproductive organ that houses babies during pregnancy, located between the bladder and rectum.

Vaginal cuff: The top of the vagina, usually sewn together front to back, after hysterectomy when the cervix is removed.

Vesicovaginal space: The area between the back wall of the bladder and front wall of the vagina.

Vulva: Female external genitalia, including the labia, clitoris, perineum, mons pubis, vaginal opening and vaginal glands.

0

References

Pathophysiology of Prolapse

1. DeLancey JOL. Fascial and muscular abnormalities in women with urethral hypermobility and anterior vaginal wall prolapse. Am J Obstet Gynecol 2002;187:93-8.

2. Otto LN, Slayden OD, Clark AL, Brenner RM. The rhesus macaque as an animal model for pelvic organ prolapse. Am J Obstet Gynecol 2002;186(3):416-21.

3. Gabriel B, Denschlag D, Gobel H, Fittkow C, Werner M, Gitsch G, Watermann D. Uterosacral ligament in postmenopausal women with or without pelvic organ prolapse. Int Urogynecol J Pelvic Floor Dysfunct 2005;16(6):475-9.

4. Clark AL, Slayden OD, Hettrich K, Brenner RM. Estrogen increases collagen I and III mRNA expression in the pelvic support tissues of the rhesus macaque. Am J Obstet Gynecol 2005;192(5):1523-9.

5. Liu YM, Choy KW, Lui WT, Pang MW, Wong YF, Yip SK. 17 beta-estradiol suppresses proliferation of fibroblasts derived from cardinal ligaments in patients with or without pelvic organ prolapse. Hum Reprod 2006;21(1):303-8.

6. Phillips CH, Anthony F, Benyon C, Monga AK. Collagen metabolism in the uterosacral ligaments and the vaginal skin of women with uterine prolapse. BJOG 2006;113(1):39-46.

7. Chung da J, Bai SW. Roles of sex steroid receptors and cell cycle regulation in pathogenesis of pelvic organ prolapse. Curr Opin Obstet Gynecol 2006;18(5):551-4.

8. Gabriel B, Watermann D, Hancke K, Gitsch G, Werner M Tempfer C, Hausen H. Increased expression of matrix metalloproteinase 2 in uterosacral ligaments is associated with pelvic organ prolapse. Int Urogynecol J Pelvic Floor Dysfunct 2006;17(5):478-82.

9. Chaliha C, Khullar V. Surgical repair of vaginal prolapse: a gynaecological hernia. Int J Surg 2006;4(4):242-50.

10. Buchsbaum GM, Duecy EE, Kerr LA, Huang LS, Perevich M, Guzick DS. Pelvic organ prolapse in nulliparous women and their parous sisters. Obstet Gynecol 2006 Dec;108(6):1388-93.

11. Larsen WI, Yavorek T. Pelvic prolapse and urinary incontinence in nulliparous college women in relation to paratrooper training. Int Urogynecol J Pelvic Floor Dysfunct 2007 Jul;18(7):769-71.

12. Delancey JO, Morgan DM, Fenner DE, Kearney DE, Guire K, Miller JM, Hussain H, Umek W, Hsu Y, Ashton-Miller JA. Comparison of levator ani muscle defects and function in women with and without pelvic organ prolapse. Obstet Gynecol 2007;109(2 pt 1):295-302.

13. Bradley CS, Zimmerman MB, Qi Y, Nygaard IE. Natural history of pelvic organ prolapse in postmenopausal women. Obstet Gynecol 2007;109(4):848-54.

14. Norton P, Allen-Brady K, Cannon-Albright L. Significant linkage evidence for a predisposition gene for pelvic floor disorders on chromosome 9. Neurourol Urodyn 2008 27(7) abstract 40.

Pelvic Organ Prolapse Incidence and Prevalence:

1. Bump RC, Norton PA. Epidemiology and natural history of pelvic floor dysfunction. Obstet Gynecol Clin North A 1998;25(4):723-46.

2. Olsen Al, Smith VJ, Bergstrom JO, Colling JC, Clark AL. Epidemiology of surgically managed pelvic organ prolapse and urinary incontinence. Obstet Gynecol 1997;89(4):501-6.

3. Luber KM, Boero S, Choe JY. The demographics of pelvic floor disorders: current observations and future projections. Am J Obstet Gynecol 2001;184(7):1496-501.

4. Lukacz ES, Lawrence JM, Buckwalter JG, Burchette RJ, Nager CW, Luber KM. Epidemiology of prolapse and incontinence questionnaire: validation of new epidemiologic survey. Int Urogynecol J Pelvic Floor Dysfunct 2005;16(4):272-84.

5. Drutz HP, Alarab M. Pelvic organ prolapse: demographics and future growth prospects. Int Urogynecol J Pelvic Floor Dysfunct 2006;17 Suppl 1:S6-9.

6. Rortveit G, Brown JS, Thom DH, Van Den Eeden SK, Creasman JM, Subak LL. Symptomatic pelvic organ prolapse: prevalence and risk factors in a population-based, racially diverse cohort. Obstet Gynecol. 2007 Jun;109(6):1396-403.

7. Nygaard I, Barber MD, Burgio KL, Kenton K, Meikle S, Schaffer J, Spino C, Whitehead WE, Wu J, Brody D: Pelvic Floor Disorders Network. Prevalence of symptomatic pelvic floor disorders in US women. JAMA 2008 Sept 17; 300(11):1311-16.

Prolapse Surgery and Sexuality:

1. Jeng CJ, Yang YC, Tzeng CR, Shen J, Wang LR. Sexual functioning after vaginal hysterectomy or transvaginal sacrospinous uterine suspension for uterine prolapse: a comparison. J Reprod Med 2005;50(9):669-74.

2. Roovers JP, van der Bom A, van Leeuwen JS, Scholten P, Heintz P, van der Vaart H. Effect of genital prolapse surgery on sexuality. J Psychosom Obstet Gynaecol 2006;2(1):43-8.

Hysterectomy and Sexuality:

1. Helstrom L, Lundberg PO, Sorbom D, Backstrom T. Sexuality after hysterectomy: a factor analysis of women's sexual lives before and after subtotal hysterectomy. Obstet Gynecol 1993;1(3):357-62.

2. Farrell SA, Kieser K. Sexuality after hysterectomy. Obstet Gynecol 2000;95(6 pt 2):1045-51.

3. Rhodes JC, Kjerulff KH, Langenberg PW, Guzinski GM. Hysterectomy and sexual functioning. JAMA 2000;283(17):2238-9.

4. Yazbeck C. Sexual function following hysterectomy. Gynecol Obstet Fertil 2004;32(1):49-54.

5. Maas CP, ter Kuile MM, Laan F, Tuijnman CC, Wijenborg PT, Trimbos JB, Kenter GG. Objective assessment of sexual arousal in women with a history of hysterectomy. BJOG 2004;111(5):456-62.

6. Maas CP, Wiejenborg PT, ter Kuile, MM. The effect of hysterectomy on sexual functioning. Annu Rev Sex Res 2004;14:83-113.

7. McPherson K, Herbert A, Judge A, Clarke A, Bridgman S, Maresh M, Overton C. Psychosexual health 5 years after hysterectomy: population-based comparison with endometrial ablation for dysfunction uterine bleeding. Health Expect 2005;8(3):234-43.

8. Parker WH, Broder MS, Liu Z, Shoupe D, Farquhar C, Berek JS. Ovarian conservation at the time of hysterectomy for benign disease. Obstet Gynecol 2005 Aug;106(2):219-26.

9. Mokate T, Wright C, Mander T. Hysterectomy and sexual function. J Br Menopause Soc 2006;12(4):153-7.

10. Ziangying H, Lili H, Yifu S. The effect of hysterectomy on ovarian blood supply an endocrine function. Climacteric 2006;9(4):283-9.

11. Teplin V, Vittinghoff E, Lin F, Learman LA, Richter HE, Kupermann M. Oophorectomy in premenopausal women: health-related quality of life and sexual functioning. Obstet Gynecol 2007;109(2 PT 1):347-54.

12. ACOG Practice Bulletin No.89. Elective and risk-reducing salpingo-oophorectomy. Obstet Gynecol. 2008 Jan; 111(1):231-41.

13. Rogers RG. Castration at the time of benign hysterectomy. The Female Patient 2008 Feb; 33:32.

14. Falcone R, Walters MD. Hysterectomy for benign disease. Obstet Gynecol 2008 Mar;111(3):753-67.

15. www.4woman.gov/faq/hysterectomy

Nonsurgical Management of Pelvic Organ Prolapse:

1. Herbison P, Plevnik S, Mantle J. Weighted vaginal cones for urinary incontinence. Cochrane Database Syst Rev 2000;(2):CD002114.

2. Hagen S, Stark D, Maher C, Adams E. Conservative management of pelvic organ prolapse in women. Cochrane Database Syst Rev 2004;(2):CD003882.

3. Hanavadi S, Durham-Hall A, Oke T, Aston N. Forgotten vaginal pessary eroding into rectum. Ann R Coll Surg Engl 2004;86(6):W18-9.

4. Jarvis SK, Hallam TK, Lujic S, Abbott JA, Vancaillie TG. Perioperative physiotherapy improves outcomes for women undergoing incontinence or prolapse surgery: results of a randomized controlled trial. Aust N Z J Obstet Gynaecol 2005;45(4):300-3.

5. Hagen S, Stark D, Maher C, Adams E. Conservative management of pelvic organ prolapse in women. Cochrane Database Syst Rev 2006;18(4):CD003882.

6. Jain A, Majoko F, Freites O. How innocent is the vaginal pessary? Two cases of vaginal cancer associated with pessary use. J Obstet Gynecol 2006;26(8):829-30.

7. Hanson LA, Schulz JA, Flood CG, Cooley B, Tam F. Vaginal pessaries in managing women wth pelvic organ prolapse and urinary incontinence: patient characteristics and factors contributing to success. Int Urogynecol J Pelvic Floor Dysfunct 2006;17(2):155-9.

8. Lukban JC, Aguirre OA, Davila GW, Sand PK Safety and effectiveness of Colpexin Sphere in the treatment of pelvic organ prolapse. Int Urogynecol J Pelvic Floor Dysfunct 2006;17(5):449-54.

Kegel:

1. Kegel AH. The physiologic treatment of poor tone and function of the genital muscles and of urinary stress incontinence. West J Surg Obstet Gynecol 1949;57(11):527-35.

2. Jones EG, Kegel AH. Treatment of urinary stress incontinence with results in 117 patients treated by active exercise of pubococcygeal. Surg Gynecol Obstet 1952;94(2):179-88.

3. Kegel AH. Sexual functions of the pubococcygeus muscle. West J Surg Obstet Gynecol 1952;60(10):521-4.

4. Kegel AH. Early genital relaxation; new technique of diagnosis and nonsurgical treatment. Obstet Gynecol 1956;8(5):545-50.

5.Graber B, Kline-Graber G. Female orgasm: role of pubococcygeus muscle. J. Clin Psychiatry 1979;40(8):348-51.

6. Messe MR, Geer JH. Voluntary vaginal musculature contractions as an enhancer of sexual arousal. Arch Sex Behav 1985;14(1):13-28.

7. Bump RC, Hurt WG, Fantl JA, Wyman JF. Assessment of Kegel pelvic muscle exercise performance after brief verbal instruction. Am J Obstet Gynecol 1991: Aug;165(2):322-7.

8. Romanzi LJ, Polaneczky M, Glazer HI. Simple test of pelvic muscle contraction during pelvic examination; correlation to surface electromyography. Neurourol Urodyn 1999;:18:603-12.

9. Cammu H, Van Nylen M, Amy JJ. A 10-year follow-up after Kegel pelvic floor muscle exercises for genuine stress incontinence. BJU Int 2000;85(6):655-8.

10. Harvey MA. Pelvic floor exercises during and after pregnancy: a systematic review of their role in preventing pelvic floor dysfunction. J Obstet Gynaecol Can 2003;25(6):487-98.

11. Beji NK, Yalcin O, Erkan HA. The effect of pelvic floor training on sexual function of treated patients. Int Urogynecol J Pelvic Floor Dysfunct 2003;14(4):234-8.

12. Dannecker C, Wolf V, Raab R, Hepp H, Anthuber C. EMG-biofeedback assisted pelvic floor muscle training is an effective therapy of stress urinary or mixed incontinence: a 7-year experience with 390 patients. Arch Gynecol Obstet 2005;273(2):3-7.

13. Bo K. Can pelvic floor muscle training prevent and treat pelvic organ prolapse? Acta Obstet Gynecol Scand 2006;85(3):263-8.

Prolapse Repair—Uterine Resuspension or Hysterectomy:

1. Thomas AG, Brodman ML, Dottino PR, Bodian C, Friedman F Jr, Bogursky E. Manchester procedure vs. vaginal hysterectomy for uterine prolapse: a comparison. J Reprod Med 1995;40(4):229-304

2. Kalogirou D, Antoniou G, Karakitsos P, Kalogirou O. Comparison of surgical and postoperative complications of vaginal hysterectomy and Manchester procedure. Eur J Gynaecol Oncol 1996;17(4):278-80.

3. Hopkins MP, Devine JB, DeLancey JO. Uterine problems discovered after presumed hysterectomy: The Manchester operation revisited. Obstet Gynecol 1997;89:846-48.

4. Shull BL, Bachofen C, Coates KW, Kuehl TJ. A transvaginal approach to repair of apical and other associated sites of pelvic organ prolapse with uterosacral ligaments. Am J Obstet Gynecol 2000;(6):1365-73.

5. Leron E, Stanton SL. Sacrohysteropexy with synthetic mesh for the management of uterovaginal prolapse. BJOG 2001;108(6):629-33.

6. Lovatsis D, Drutz HP. Safety and efficacy of sacrospinous vault suspension. Int Urogynecol J Pelvic Floor Dysfunct 2002;13(5):308-13.

7. Elghorori MR, Ahmed AA, Sadhukhan M, Al-Taher H. Vaginal sacrospinous fixation: experience in a district general hospital. J. Obstet Gynaecol 2002;22(6):658-62.

8. van Brummen HJ, van de Pol G, Aalders CI, Heintz AP, van der Vaart CH. Sacrospinous hysteropexy compared to vaginal hysterectomy as primary surgical treatment for descensus uteri: effects on urinary symptoms. Int Urogynecol J Pelvic Floor Dysfunct 2003;14(5):350-5.

9. Barranger E, Fritel X, Pigne A. Abdominal sacrohysteropexy in young women with uterovaginal prolapse: long-term follow-up. Am J Obstet Gynecol 2003;189(5):1245-50

10. Tyagi R, Romanzi LJ. Uterine preservation and the repair of apical prolapse: a comparison of transvaginal surgical outcomes for apical pelvic organ prolapse with and without hysterectomy. AUGS joint scientific meeting, 2004; and SUFU joint scientific meeting, 2004. (Abstracts).

11. Ng CC, Han WH. Comparison of effectiveness of vaginal and abdominal routes in treatment of severe uterovaginal or vault prolapse. Singapore Med J 2004;45(10):475-81.

12. Limb J, Wood K, Weinberger M, Miyazaki F, Aboseif S. Sacrocolpopexy using mersilene mesh in the treatment of vaginal vault prolapse. World J Urol 2005;23(1):55-60.

13. Elneil S, Cutner AS, Remy M, Lether AT, Toozs-Hobson P, Wise B. Abdominal sacrocolpopexy for vault prolapse without burial of mesh: a case series. BJOG 2005;112(4):486-9.

14. Lo TS, Horng SG, Huang HJ, Lee SJ, Liang CC. Repair of recurrent vaginal vault prolapse using sacrospinous ligament fixation with mesh interposition and reinforcement. Acta Obstet Gynecol Scand 2005;84(10):992-5.

15. Allahdin S, Herd D, Reid BA. Twenty-five sarospinous ligament fixation procedures in a district general hospital: our experience. J Obstet Gynaecol 2005;25(4):361-3.

16. Ross JW, Preston M. Laparoscopic sacrocolpopexy for severe vaginal vault prolapse: five-year outcome. J Minim Invasive Gynecol 2005;12(3):221-6.

17. Ayhan A, Esin S, Guven S, Salman C, Ozyuncu O. The Manchester operation for uterine prolapse. Int J Gynaecol Obstet 2006;92(3):228-33.

18. Skiadas CC, Godstein DP, Laufer MR. The Manchester-Fothergill procedure as a fertility sparing alternative for pelvic organ prolapse in young women. J Pediatr Adolesc Gynecol 2006;19(2):89-93.

19. Silva WA, Pauls RN, Segal JL, Rooney CM, Kleeman SD, Karram MM. Uterosacral ligament vault suspension: five year outcomes. Obstet Gynecol 2006;108(2):255-63.

20. Demirci F, Ozdemir I, Somunkiran A, Doyran GD, Alhan A, Gul B. Abdominal sacrohysterpexy in young women with uterovaginal prolapse: results of 20 cases. J Reprod Med 2006;51(7):539-43.

21. Diwan A, Rardin CR, Strohsnitter WC, Weld A, Rosenblatt P, Kohli N. Laparoscopic uterosacral ligament uterine suspension compared with vaginal hysterectomy with vaginal vault suspension for uterovaginal prolapse. Int Urogynecol J Pelvic Floor Dysfunct 2006;17(1):79-83.

22. Demirci F, Ozdemir I, Somunkiran A, Topuz S, Ivibozkurt C, Duras Doyran G, Kemik Gul O. Perioperative complications in abdominal sacrocolpopexy and vaginal sacrospinous ligament fixation procedures. Int Urogyn J Pelvic Floor Dysfunct 2007;18(3):257-61.

23. Maher C, Baessler K, Glazener CM, Adams EJ, Hagen S. Surgical management of pelvic organ prolapse in women. Cochrane Database Syst Rev 2007;18(3):CD004014.

24. Schwartz M, Abbott KR, Glazerman L, Soloewski C, Jarnagin B, Ailawadi R, Lucente V. Positive symptom improvement with laparoscopic uterosacral ligament repair for uterine or vaginal vault prolapse: interim results from an active multicenter trial. J Minim Invasive Gynecol. 2007;14(5):570-6.

25. Jha S, Moran PA. National survey on the management of prolapse in the UK. Neurourol Urodyn 2007;26(3):325-31.

26. Committee on Gynecologic Practice, ACOG. ACOG Committee Opinion no. 85: Pelvic Organ Prolapse. Obstet Gynecol 2007;110(3):17-29.

27. Denman MA, Gregory WT, Boyles SH, Smith V, Edwards SR, Clark AL. Reoperation 10 years after surgically managed pelvic organ prolapse and urinary incontinence. Am J Obstet Gynecol. 2008 May;198(5):555.

Prolapse Repair—Graft Materials

1. Puccio F, Solazzo M, Marciano P.Comparison of three different mesh materials in tension-free inguinal hernia repair: prolene versus vypro versus surgisis. Int Surg. 2005 Jul-Aug;90(3 Suppl):S21-3.

2. Davila GW, Drutz H, Deprest J. Clinical implications of the biology of grafts. Conclusions of the 2005 IUGA grafts roundtable. Int Urogynecol Pelvic Floor Dysfunct. 2006 Jun:17 Suppl 1:S51-5.

3. Edelman DS, Selesnick H."Sports" hernia: treatment with biologic mesh (Surgisis): a preliminary study. Surg Endosc. 2006 Jun;20(6):971-3.

4 Chen CC, Ridgeway B, Paraiso MF. Biologic grafts and synthetic meshes in pelvic reconstructive surgery. Clin Obstet Gynecol. 2007 Jun;50(2):383-411. Review

5. Ansaloni L, Cambrini P, Catena F, Di Saverio S, Gagliardi S, Gazzotti F, Hodde JP, Metzger DW, D'Alessandro L, Pinna AD.Immune response to small intestinal submucosa (surgisis) implant in humans: preliminary observations.J Invest Surg. 2007 Jul-Aug;20(4):237-41

6 Jacobs M, Gomez E, Plasencia G, Lopez-Penalver C, Lujan H, Velarde D, Jessee T.Use of surgisis mesh in laparoscopic repair of hiatal hernias.Surg Laparosc Endosc Percutan Tech. 2007 Oct;17(5):365-8.

7 Jakus SM, Shapiro A, Hall CD.Biologic and synthetic graft use in pelvic surgery: a review.Obstet Gynecol Surv. 2008 Apr;63(4):253-66. Review.

8. Ayubi FS, Armstrong PJ, Mattia MS, Parker DM. Abdominal wall hernia repair: a comparison of Permacol and Surgisis grafts in a rat hernia model. Hernia. 2008 Aug;12(4):373-8.

9. Jia X, Glazener C, Mowatt G, MacLennan G, Bain C, Fraser C, Burr J. Efficacy and safety of using mesh or grafts in surgery for anterior and/or posterior vaginal wall prolapse: systematic review and meta-analysis. BJOG. 2008 Oct;115(11):1350-61

10. www.nice/org/uk, IPG267 Surgical repair of vaginal wall prolapse using mesh: guidance

11. www.fda.gov/cdrh/safety/102008-surgicalmesh.html.

12. www.fda.gov/cdrh/consumer/surgicalmesh-popsui.html

Prolapse and Bladder:

1. White GR: Cystocele: a radical cure by suturing lateral sulci of vagina to white line of pelvic fascia. JAMA 1909;21:1707-10.

2. Borstad E, Rud T. The risk of developing urinary stress incontinence after vaginal repair in continent women. Acta Obstet Gynecol Scan 1989;68:545-49.

3. Romanzi LJ, Chaikin D, Blaivas JG. Effect of vaginal prolapse on voiding J Urol 1999;161:581-586.

4. Fitzgerald MP, Kulkarni N, Fenner D. Postoperative resolution of urinary retention in patients with advanced pelvic organ prolapse. Am J Obstet Gynecol 2000;183:1261-64.

5. Weber AM, Walters MD, Piedmonte MR, Ballard LA. Anterior colporraphy: a randomized trial of three surgical techniques. Am J Obstet Gynecol 2001;185: 1299-1306.

6. Huebner M, Hsu Y, Fenner DE. The use of graft materials in vaginal pelvic floor surgery. Int J Gynaecol Obstet 2006;92(3):279-88.

7. Pulliam SJ, Ferzandi TR, Hota LS, Elkadry EA, Rosenblatt PL. Use of synthetic mesh in pelvic reconstructive surgery: a survey of attitudes and practice patterns of urogynecologists. Int Urogynecol J Pelvic Floor Dysfunct 2007;18(12):1405-8.

Prolapse and Rectum:

1. Abramov Y, Gandhi S, Goldberg RP, Botros SM, Kwon C, Sand PK. Site-specific rectocele repair compared with standard posterior colporrhaphy. Obstet Gynecol. 2005;105(2):314-8.

2. Paraiso MF, Barber MD, Muir TW, Walters MD. Rectocele repair: a randomized trial of three surgical techniques including graft augmentation. Am J Obstet Gynecol. 2006;195(6):1762-71.

3. Gustilo-Ashby AM, Paraiso MF, Jelovsek JE, Walters MD, Barber MD. Bowel symptoms 1 year after surgery for prolapse: further analysis of a randomized trial of rectocele repair. Am J Obstet Gynecol 2007;197(1):76, e1-5.

Vaginal Laxity and Vaginal Rejuvenation:

1. Rovner ES, Ginsberg DA. Posterior vaginal wall prolapse: transvaginal repair of pelvic floor relaxation, rectocele, and perineal laxity. Tech Urol 2001 Jun;7(2):161-8.

2. Fox JC, Fletcher JG, Zinsmeister AR, Seide B, Riederer SJ, Bharucha AE. Effect of aging on anorectal and pelvic floor functions in females. Dis Colon Rectum 2006;49(11):1726-35.

3. Pardo JS, Solà VD, Ricci PA, Guiloff EF, Freundlich OK. Colpoperineoplasty in women with a sensation of a wide vagina. Acta Obstet Gynecol Scand 2006;85(9):1125-7.

4. Committee on Gynecologic Practice, ACOG. ACOG Committee Opinion no 378: Vaginal "rejuvenation" and cosmetic vaginal procedures. Obstet Gynecol 2007 Sep;110(3):737-8.

Urinary Incontinence:

1. Romanzi LJ. Management of the urethral outlet in patients with severe prolapse. Curr Opin Urol 2002;12(4):339-44.

2. Stewart WF, Van Rooyen JB, Cundiff GW, Abrams P, Herzog AR, Corey R, Hunt TL, Wein AJ. Prevalence and burden of overactive bladder in the United States. World J Urol 2003;20(6):327-36.

3. Coyne KS, Zhou Z, Thompson C, Versi E. The impact on health-related quality of life of stress, urge and mixed urinary incontinence. BJU Int 2003;92(7):731-5.

4. Shah DK, Paul EM, Amukele S, Eisenberg ER, Badlani GH. Broad based tension-free synthetic sling for stress urinary incontinence: 5-year outcome. J Urol 2003;170(3):849-51.

5. Romanzi LJ. Pathophysiology of overactive bladder and its pharmacologic management. Manag Care Interface 2005;18 Suppl B:10-5.

6. Jeon MJ, Chung da J, Park JH, Kim SK, Kim JW, Bai SW. Surgical therapeutic index of tension-free vaginal tape and transobturator tape for stress urinary incontinence. Gynecol Obstet Invest 2008;65(1):41-6.

Wound Healing:

1. Ashcroft GS, Dodsworth J, van Boxtel E, Tarnuzzer RW, Horan MA, Schultz GS, Ferguson MW. Estrogen accelerates cutaneous wound healing associated with increase in TGF-beta1 levels. Nat Med 1997;3(11):1209-15.

2. Ashcroft GS, Greenwell-Wild T, Horan MA, Wahl SM, Ferguson MW. Topical estrogen accelerates cutaneous wound healing in aged humans associated with an altered inflammatory response. Am J Pathol 1999;155(4):1137-46.

3. Dal Lago A, De Martini D, Flore R, Gaetani E, Gasbarrini A, Gerardino L, Pola R, Santoloquido A, Serricchio M, Tondi P, Nolfe G. Effects of propionyl-L-carnitine on peripheral arterial obliterative disease of the lower limbs: a double-blind clinical trial. Drugs Exp Clin Res 1999;25(1):29-36.

4. Hart AM, Wiberg M, Youle M, Terenghi G. Systemic acetyl-L-carnitine eliminates sensory neuronal loss after peripheral axotomy: a new clinical approach in the management of peripheral nerve trauma. Exp Brain Res 2002;145(2):182-9.

5. Witte MB, Barbul A. Arginine physiology and its implication for wound healing. Wound Repair Regen 2003;11(6):419-23.

6. Desneves KJ, Todorovic BE, Cassar A, Crowe TC. Treatment with supplementary arginine, vitamin C and zinc in patients with pressure ulcers: a randomised controlled trial. Clin Nutr 2005;24(6):979-87.

7. Arslan E, Basterzi Y, Aksoy A, Majka C, Unal S, Sari A, Demirkan F. The additive effects of carnitine and ascorbic acid on distally burned dorsal skin flap in rats. Med Sci Monit 2005;11(6):BR176-180.

8. Stechmiller JK, Childress B, Cowan L. Arginine supplementation and wound healing. Nutr Clin Pract 2005;20(1):52-61.

9. Raschke M, Rasmussen MH, Govender S, Segal D, Suntum M, Christiansen JS. Effects of growth hormone in patients with tibial fracture: a randomized, double-blind, placebo-controlled clinical trial. Eur J Endocrinol 2007;156(3):341-51.

Historical:

1. J . Marion Sims:
http://en.wikipedia.org/wiki/J._Marion_Sims

2. Arnold Kegel: http://en.wikipedia.org/wiki/Arnold_Kegel
http://en.wikipedia.org/wiki/Kegel_exercise

3. Hernia Truss: http://herniarelievers.com
http://alphabrace.com

4. Life expectancy: www.cdc.gov/nchs/nvss.htm
www.efmoody.com/estate/lifeexpectancy.html
www.oheschools.org
www.statistics.gov.uk

5. Anesthesia:
http://neurosurgery.mgh.harvard.edu/history/ether1.htm

6. Shokeir AA, Hussein MI. The urology of pharaonic Egypt-historical review. BJU Int 1999 Nov; 84(7):755-61.

Appendix

5 Second Kegel Score Test				
	0	1	2	3
Pressure	None	Weak	Moderate	Strong
Duration	None	<1 Second	1-5 Seconds	>5 Seconds
Displacement	None	Slight Rotation	Full Rotation	Gripped

Your Score: ________/9

Instructions for the Examining Clinician[1]

During the bimanual portion of the gynecologic checkup, evaluate the pressure, duration and vaginal axis displacement generated by the patient during Kegel contraction of the levator ani muscles as follows:

Pressure:

Weak—a flicker-like contraction that generates minimal or no resistance around examining fingers
Moderate—definite but unsustainable resistance
Strong—sustained resistance to examining fingers

Duration:

Evaluate baseline tone before Kegel effort. Record the time of maximal Kegel contraction effort from initiation to return to baseline tone: none, <1 second, 1-5 seconds, >5 seconds

Displacement:

With exam fingertips applied to the anterior vaginal wall, evaluate the vaginal axis during Kegel as fingers are elevated caudad and rotated anteriorly as follows:

Slight—elevation/rotation distal exam fingers only
Whole—elevation/rotation full length, no overriding fingers
Gripped—elevation/rotation of full length that does cause fingers to override

1 Romanzi LJ, Polaneczky M, Glazer HI. Simple test of pelvic muscle contraction during pelvic examination; correlation to surface electromyography. Neurourol Urodyn 1999;18:603-12.

Information Resources

1. American College of Obstetrics and Gynecology: www.acog.org
2. American Urogynecologic Society: www.augs.org
3. American Urologic Association: www.urologyhealth.org
4. HYSTERSISTERS: www.hystersisters.com
5. International Urogynecological Association: www.iuga.org (see urogynecology information)
6. National Association For Continence: www.nafc.org
7. National Women's Health Information Center:
   www.4woman.gov
   1.800.994.9662
   TDD: 1.888.220.5446
8. Society of Gynecologic Surgeons www.sgsonline.org
9. Society for Urodynamics and Female Urology: www.sufuorg.com

Index

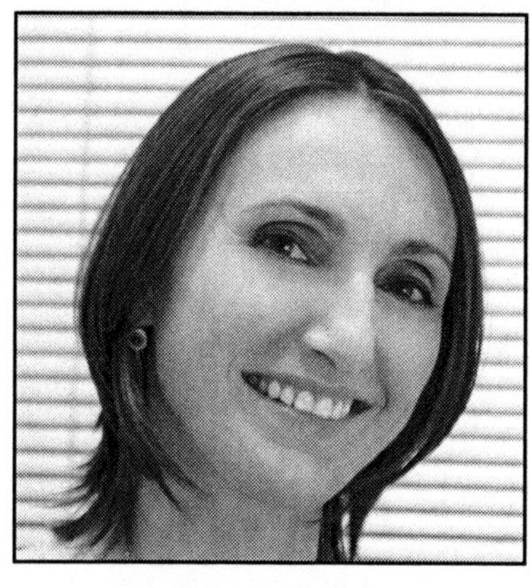

Lauri Romanzi is a world-renowned reconstructive pelvic surgeon and urogynecologist. She is an Associate Professor of Obstetrics and Gynecology at New York Presbyterian Hospital-Weill Cornell Medical College. She serves on the fistula subcommittee of the International Urogynecology Association, is a charter member of the Society of International Humanitarian Surgeons, reviews submissions for several respected medical journals and serves on the Editorial Advisory Board of the Journal of Gender Specific Medicine.

Dr. Romanzi is the pioneer of a scar-free, uterus-preserving (no hysterectomy) technique of uterine prolapse repair and was the first surgeon in Manhattan to perform minimally invasive sling procedure for urinary incontinence.

Her charitable works include volunteer fistula repair surgery with the International Organization for Women and Development in Niger, serving as visiting professor at Kilimanjaro Christian Medical Center in Tanzania, and performing reconstructive surgery and fistula repair at Panzi Hospital in the Democratic Republic of Congo through Harvard Humanitarian Initiative's program to relieve human suffering in war and disaster.

Dr. Romanzi has two children in college and lives and works in Manhattan.

LaVergne, TN USA
24 May 2010
183786LV00004B/69/P